STOPPNow:
(Stop the Organized Pill Pushers) Now

by

Janet Colbert

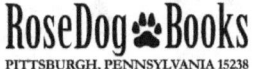

PITTSBURGH, PENNSYLVANIA 15238

The contents of this work including, but not limited to, the accuracy of events, people, and places depicted; opinions expressed; permission to use previously published materials included; and any advice given or actions advocated are solely the responsibility of the author, who assumes all liability for said work and indemnifies the publisher against any claims stemming from publication of the work.

All Rights Reserved
Copyright © 2017 by Janet Colbert

No part of this book may be reproduced or transmitted, downloaded, distributed, reverse engineered, or stored in or introduced into any information storage and retrieval system, in any form or by any means, including photocopying and recording, whether electronic or mechanical, now known or hereinafter invented without permission in writing from the publisher or copyright owner.

RoseDog Books
585 Alpha Drive, Suite 103
Pittsburgh, PA 15238
Visit our website at *www.rosedogbookstore.com*

ISBN: 978-1-4809-7562-0
eISBN: 978-1-4809-7585-9

This book is dedicated to all the parents who have lost their children. My heart is broken for you and for them.

DISCLAIMER

This book is based on facts. The trial and my correspondence with legislators occurred as reported here. Great care was taken to report them as they transpired.

ACKNOWLEDGEMENTS AND RESOURCES

All that is necessary for evil to triumph is for good men to do nothing.

– Edmund Burke

Many people we have met along this journey have reached out to offer their help.

Tom Shea, of All Graphics Impressions, Inc., www.agimpressionsinc.com, introduced himself to us at an event where we were speaking. He offered to make us a STOPPNow banner at no charge. He has also printed business cards for us either at cost or at no charge. Most of all, Tom has encouraged us, understanding both what we are trying to accomplish and the importance of our mission.

Anthony Reinosa lost a good friend to the epidemic. Before Anthony contacted us, I had been working on the website myself – and it showed. Anthony improved the site for us and continues to update it as needed. I am grateful to him for his technical support.

My dear friend Roberta came to protests right from work – in her office attire, including heels. I would tell her to keep sneakers in her car. She purchased STOPPNow flags and STOPPNow umbrellas, which we use when we are protesting either in the blazing sun or in the pouring rain. Roberta is just one of many who make me wish I could take all the pain away from the parents who have suffered this terrible, needless loss.

I am grateful to **my editor, Jamie Morris.** What a blessing that she started this process not knowing anything about the prescription drug epidemic or a pill mill, because she needed me to explain everything clearly and forced me to be concise. I am a much better writer because of her.

There are many other advocacy groups and good people who I would like to recognize for trying to put an end to the epidemic:

Feduprally.org – Fed Up! Rally for a Federal Response to The Opioid Epidemic.

Andrew Kolodny, M.D.
Co-Director, Opioid Policy Research Institute for Behavioral Health
Schneider Institutes for Health Policy,
Heller School for Social Policy & Management
Brandeis University

Jim Hall, Epidemiologist
ARSH Center for Applied Research on Substance Use and Health Disparities
Nova Southeastern University

Steeredstraight.org – Michael R. DeLeon

Learn2Cope.org – Joanne Peterson

Maureen Kielian – mkielian@aol.com

And, of course, we are **STOPPNow**. Join us. We need a louder voice to affect change.

STOPPNow.com – See "current projects" to learn how you can be part of the solution.

Email me, **Janet Colbert, STOPPNow Florida** – stoppnow@yahoo.com, to let me know what successes you're seeing in your state and your thoughts on the book.

Emily Walden, STOPPNow Kentucky – ewalden3@gmail.com

CONTENTS

INTRODUCTION xi
CHAPTER ONE: Why STOPPNow was formed .1
CHAPTER TWO: Renee 5
CHAPTER THREE: The Effects 9
CHAPTER FOUR: The Cause 21
CHAPTER FIVE: Politicians 29
CHAPTER SIX: Senator Eleanor Sobel 43
CHAPTER SEVEN: The Taking Down of Joel Shumrak 47
CHAPTER EIGHT: Legislation Needed: Is Anyone Listening? 57
CHAPTER NINE: Still Work to Be Done 63
CHAPTER TEN: We Just Don't Know When To Give Up 71
CHAPTER ELEVEN: Carol 77
CHAPTER TWELVE: Smoke and Mirrors: 81
CHAPTER THIRTEEN: More Smoke, More Mirrors 91
CHAPTER FOURTEEN: Yet Another Meeting 103
CHAPTER FIFTEEN: Law Enforcement and DEA Is All We Have . . .109
CHAPTER SIXTEEN: First Degree Murder Charge:
State vs. Dr. Gerald J. Klein 111
EPILOGUE 297
APPENDIX A: CDC Guideline for Prescribing Opioids
for Chronic Pain, 2016 313
APPENDIX B: Letter from the U.S. Surgeon General 317

INTRODUCTION

Let me start this book about the prescription-pill epidemic by introducing you to the term "pill mill," as described on Florida Attorney General Pam Bondi's website, http://www.myfloridalegal.com.

Pill Mill Initiative

What are Pill Mills?

A "pill mill" is a doctor's office, clinic, or health care facility that routinely conspires in the prescribing and dispensing of controlled substances outside the scope of the prevailing standards of medical practice in the community or violates the laws of the state of Florida regarding the prescribing or dispensing of controlled prescription drugs.

Issue

In 2010, Florida led the nation in diverted prescription drugs, resulting in seven Floridians dying every day and countless others throughout the nation. Our state had become the destination for distributors and abusers through the proliferation of pill mills.

While legitimate pain-management clinics do exist to serve those with chronic pain or terminal illness, other unscrupulous clinics, called pill mills, merely serve as drug traffickers. Common characteristics of pill mills include: cash-only/no insurance; no appointments; armed guards; little or no medical records; grossly inadequate physical examinations; and large prescription doses of narcotics that exceed the boundaries of acceptable medical care.

The Facts

The Centers for Disease Control and Prevention has declared prescription drug abuse an epidemic in America.

Florida was the epicenter of prescription drug diversion because – until recently – our state had weak regulatory oversight of pain management practices, limited oversight of physician dispensing habits, and no statewide Prescription Drug Monitoring Program (PDMP).

In 2010, pharmaceutical drug diversion meant an average of seven Floridians dying a day due to prescription drug overdoses.

In 2010, there were more than 900 registered pain management clinics in Florida, but as of January 2014, there were 367 registered pain management clinics in Florida.

Florida's dubious distinction as the 'epicenter' of the nation's 'pill mill' epidemic was solidified in 2010 when DEA's Automation of Reports and Consolidated Orders System (ARCOS) reported that ninety-eight of the top 100 oxycodone dispensing physicians in the nation were located in Florida. Today, none of the top 100 dispensing physicians reside in Florida.

2011 Anti-Pill Mill Bill

Attorney General Bondi worked with the Florida Legislature to pass legislation cracking down on Florida's pill mills.

I have spoken to many who believe the pill-mill epidemic is over in Florida. The final statement above, while true, is misleading, and it contributes to that misconception. Florida did pass legislation that outlawed physicians from dispensing narcotics directly from their office in 2010.

But the same physicians who dispensed the narcotics are still here. The only difference now is that they write prescriptions, rather than dispensing directly. These physicians have a license to kill. The Board of Medicine could revoke the license of every high prescribing drug dealer doctor, but, instead, every year the deaths from prescription opiates increase. And the numbers of babies born into the hellish world of opiate addiction continues to increase as well.

You see, Florida's dirty little secret is well known to those who could have stopped this life-destroying epidemic but didn't. What would be required to halt the deluge of prescription-pill related deaths? Strong leadership guided by a solid moral compass. However, as you will see, the lack of such qualities in our elected officials has allowed the opiate epidemic to escalate.

CHAPTER ONE

Why STOPPNow Was Formed

I first became aware of the prescription drug epidemic while working as a neonatal intensive care nurse on a very busy unit located in Broward County, Florida. The conversation in the nurses' lounge every day focused on why, all of a sudden, in 2009 we had so many drug-addicted babies on our unit. Both the number of babies we were seeing as well as the extent of their suffering was the worst we had ever seen. In the past, we might have seen an occasional newborn addicted to cocaine **(illegal drug)**, but nothing like this.

Now in 2009 at our children's hospital (a sixty-bed unit) we were admitting on a consistent basis babies suffering from drug withdrawal. The drug these babies were all testing positive for was the opiate, oxycodone (legal drug). Pain pills.

On one particular morning, while holding a screaming Baby J and talking on the phone with his mother, I, who normally am able to compose myself while speaking to a mother, had to struggle not to explode. She asked, so casually, as if she were not involved at all, "How's Baby J?"

"He's screaming right now," I said. "Can't you hear him?"

Her only response was to ask why he was screaming. And then I said it: "Because he's suffering from drug withdrawal."

As if I hadn't even spoken, all she said was, "Is he hungry?"

Baby J had already been on our unit for months at this time. We had been treating him with morphine and phenobarbital every three hours to help him through the suffering. He trembled so much he was unable to form the negative pressure needed to suck from a bottle. He was in an almost-constant frenzy and slept very little.

But why? Why were Baby J and so many other infants suddenly arriving into the world with drug addictions? It wasn't long before I discovered the cause of this epidemic – and learned that Broward County, Florida, was the epicenter.

STOPPNow

Exhibit 1

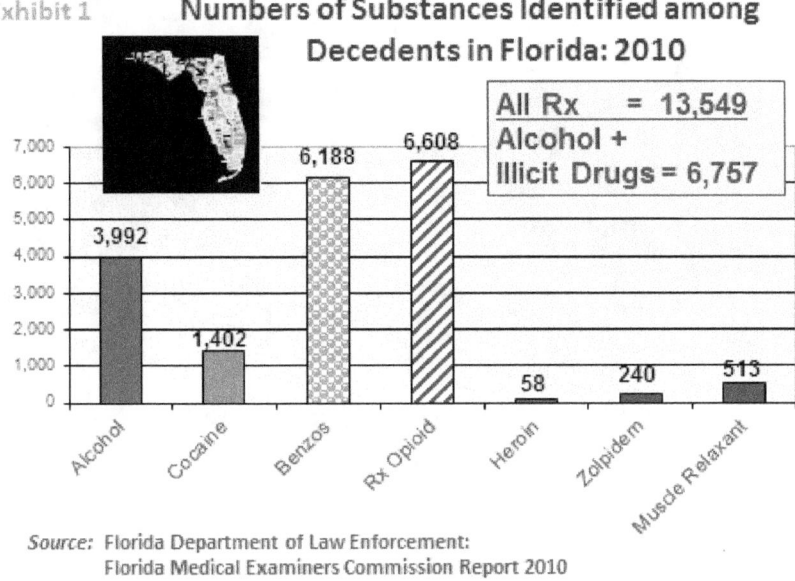

Source: Florida Department of Law Enforcement:
Florida Medical Examiners Commission Report 2010

Courtesy of Jim Hall, Epidemiologist, Nova University
Important to note in 2010: Opioid deaths 6,608; Heroin 58

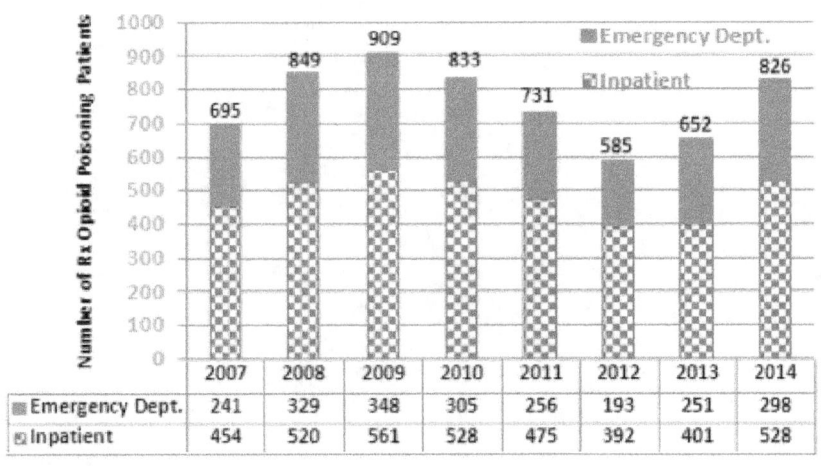

Source: Analysis of data from the Florida Agency for Health Care Administration

CHAPTER TWO

Renee

My children grew up in a neighborhood with lots of other kids. They played on baseball teams, starting with t-ball when they were very young, so our family spent many evenings at the ballpark. I would rush home from work, and we would hurriedly eat dinner to make it to the game – where all the parents would sit in the bleachers, cheering the kids on.

Renee and I met through our children. She lived in the last house on our block and had four boys. They gave her a run for her money. Blayne was her third of four. He had an angelic face, set with the biggest brown eyes you ever saw and framed with curly blond locks. One day, while my parents were babysitting my children, my mom answered the door to find innocent little four-year old Blayne standing there. Blayne asked, "Where's Diegle live?" (Diegle's house was the neighborhood hangout for the older children, those who were allowed to venture onto the next block.)

My mother brought Blayne into the house, saying, "Never mind where Diegle lives!" and called Renee. It seems that Blayne had gotten up from his nap and headed off on his own, when Renee's back was turned. Renee was frantic and had all the immediate neighbors combing the neighborhood looking for him.

Many years have passed since that day, and over the course of them, Blayne only became a bigger and bigger challenge – finally becoming a drug user. Renee tried helping him – she tried the tough-love approach with him. But no matter how much she and her husband had tried to help Blayne, he would go right back to the drugs. Finally, Renee received a phone call in November of 2009 from the hospital telling her that Blayne had overdosed. Renee rushed to his bedside to tell him she loved him. During that conversation, Blayne, told his mother about the "pain clinics" springing up in Broward County. He explained that one could just go in feigning an injury and walk out with a stash of drugs. (We later learned these clinics typically dispensed three specific drugs: oxycodone, an opiate; Xanax, for anti-anxiety; and Soma, a muscle relaxer – with each customer receiving all three and always in exorbitant amounts.)

Renee pleaded with the hospital to help her son with his addiction, but the answer to her pleas was that there were no available treatment beds, and the hospital released Blayne. Just two weeks later, when Blayne's brother Cory presented Renee with a healthy baby grandchild, Renee, elated and feeling that maybe this new child was a harbinger of change for the better, went to visit her newborn grandson. Then, on her way home from the hospital, just as dusk was falling, she was caught in a traffic jam. Police were directing cars around an accident. As she passed the accident scene, Renee saw a body bag lying off to the side of the road – and a little after midnight that night, Renee was awakened by the Broward Sheriff's office. They were sorry, but they were there to notify her of her son Blayne's death. Blayne died in the accident that Renee passed earlier in the evening. Blayne was in the body bag that Renee saw lying on the side of the road.

Blayne was killed just three miles from the hospital where his nephew had just been born. No one knows for sure if that's where he was headed, and the officers could not explain exactly what had happened. It seems that Blayne had been walking along State Road 7, and he either walked in front of the car, or the car veered off the roadway and hit him. While Renee never learned how, precisely, her son was killed, she did explain to the officers that night that her son was struggling with drug addiction. When she told them about the pain clinics he'd mentioned to her and explained that they were the ones supplying the drugs to him, the officers nodded. They knew all about the clinics.

Soon after Blayne's death, Renee asked me if I would help her write letters to see if we could do something about closing the clinics. At the time, we had no idea just how big this task was going to be. It turns out the pain clinic owners, many of whom are former felons, had an ingenious plan: they found a way to deal drugs legally. They start by getting a letter of occupancy from the city or county. Then they find a doctor willing to become, in essence, a drug dealer and dispense the drugs onsite.

Then many of those to whom they dispensed the drugs go on to sell what they don't take themselves. For instance, the father of Baby J, the drug-addicted baby I spoke of earlier, didn't consume all the pills he was given. He, like so many others that frequented the clinics, left the clinic with so many pills that he was able to sell what he wasn't taking. When he was arrested, also like so many others, he would call to check on his baby from jail. You see, the police were arresting those the clinic owners made into little drug-dealing entrepreneurs – those they had made into drug addicts. While the real drug dealers, the big-time dealers, remained untouched inside the buildings. In fact, I've been told by some that organized crime was involved and that I was going to get killed doing this.

Which brings us to STOPPNow. I based the name of the organization on what we were trying to accomplish – the cessation of the pill-mill industry. The original name was STOPP ("Stop the Organized Pill Pushers). When we tried to secure the name for a web page, however, we found we had to add "Now," as the domain name "Stopp" was already taken. Unfortunately, "now" is taking a very long time. What we wanted was to find someone who would care enough to stop the deaths. But when we saw that our letters were not accomplishing what we naively thought they would, we started holding peaceful protests in front of the pain clinics (pill mills). Our first peaceful protest was held on August 24, 2010, at The Pain Relief Center, 3088 Griffin Road Fort, Lauderdale, Florida.

At our protests, local residents and those from neighborhood businesses would come up to tell us about the syringes they found all over the parking lots and surrounding yards. Parents who had lost their children would drive by and stop in the middle of the six-lane highway with tears streaming down their faces to tell us about their buried child. Soon, people from all over the country began writing to us, pouring out their hearts, telling us of their loved ones lost while no one listened or cared. We started a dedication page on our website.

There, we posted pictures of children, siblings, and spouses lost to this prescription-pill epidemic. The destruction to the community and the devastation endured by so many families are preventable. And that is our goal.

CHAPTER THREE

The Effects

In an article titled, "Three Broward women join forces to fight oxycodone trade," which appeared in the *Sun Sentinel* on September 17, 2010, Tonya Alanez explained our attempts to halt the pill mills. Just five days later, we received an email from a pediatrician that showed us clearly how those dying from prescription drugs were not just "somebody else's" kids. The problem is affecting our entire society.

From: Wright, John

To: Stoppnow@yahoo.com

Date: September 22, 2010

Kudos on your efforts to eradicate the pain clinics in Broward County!!! I am a native of Fort Lauderdale, a pediatrician, and the medical director of the Broward County Child Protection Team (CPT). I have a special interest in child abuse pediatrics and was recently board certified in this new specialty from the American Board of Medical Specialties. As part of my responsibilities to CPT, I review all the child abuse allegations that are reported in Broward County, approximately 20,000 per year. You would be amazed at how many of these are associated with prescription drug abuse in the parent or guardian. I am fully supportive of your efforts as a citizen, doctor, child abuse pediatrician, and parent of four children.

If there is anything I can do, please do not hesitate to contact me.

Sincerely,

John E. Wright, M.D., FAAP

From: Stoppnow@yahoo.com

To: Wright, John

Dr. Wright:

Thank you very much for your interest. The response from the public has been overwhelming. Channel 7 was interested in doing a documentary. They were at our first rally. The drug-addicted baby would give them a new aspect on the problem to keep the story alive. I am a neonatal intensive care nurse and this is one of the reasons I have started this organization. May I forward your email to Carmel Cafiero?

The politicians have to this point sent me nice letters in response to my pleas to them but are doing nothing to close the pain clinics. When the public outcry is loud enough to cost them an election, perhaps they'll listen.

Respectfully,

Janet Colbert

We often had county commissioners from Broward and Fort Lauderdale join us to protest. Our politicians on a state and national level, however, could not be moved to use their positions to put this fire out. To this day, no official has lost public office due to inaction in response to this epidemic. In fact, it may be that the opposite has occurred and that the loss of position has been to the very few who tried to shed light on this national holocaust.

The hospital I worked for did not like what I was doing. I was told that they didn't want their paying customers to know that there were drug-addicted babies on our unit. My response was that every hospital in Broward County has babies born addicted to drugs. This crisis has spread in our state and in our country. St. Joseph's Hospital in Tampa took a different view on the crisis. St. Joseph's reported that thirty percent of babies born at their facility were born addicted to these drugs. One of the doctors from St. Joseph's Women's Hospital in Tampa was part of the Statewide Task Force on Prescription Drug Abuse and Newborns formed by Attorney General Pam Bondi in 2012.

The tragedy of ignoring this situation is made clear in the second email I received from Dr. Wright:

From Wright, John

Date: September 23, 2010

To: Stoppnow@yahoo.com

Here are some more researched figures. In the past three years, Broward County has initiated investigations or reviewed maltreatment allegations on an average of 13,000 per year (13,042 in 2009). It is estimated that each of these reports refers to 2-2.5 children. Each report has on average two reported maltreatments. From my review (the computer doesn't record this specifically), allegations of prescription drug abuse are present in about one-third of these reports. When we actually do investigate the cases, we find that one or more caretakers are using prescription pain medication in even more cases than are reported. I would say that prescription drug abuse is one of the leading drivers of child maltreatment in our community.

John E. Wright, M.D., FAAP

The information shared by Dr. Wright in his email describes the tragedy of children being raised in homes by drug-addicted caregivers (parents or otherwise). But, as is the case with Baby J, there are victims of the prescription-drug epidemic who are so young – newborns – that pediatricians such as Dr. Wright would not even have had the opportunity to attend them. The following comes from Florida Attorney General Pam Bondi's website:

PRESCRIPTION DRUG ABUSE AND NEWBORNS

Neonatal Abstinence Syndrome

Neonatal Abstinence Syndrome (NAS) refers to a group of medical complications associated with the withdrawal process newborns typically experience after birth if their mothers have used addictive illicit or prescription drugs during pregnancy. Florida is seeing a growing number NAS cases and these babies are born suffering from withdrawal symptoms such as tremors, seizures, abdominal pain, incessant crying, and rapid breathing. In 2011, there were 1,563 instances of newborns diagnosed with drug exposure in Florida, a three-fold increase since 2007.

A study published by the *Journal of the American Medical Association* in April 2012 shows that, nationally, the number of babies born exposed to prescription drugs has nearly tripled in the past decade.

In 2012 Florida Legislature recognized the problem and adopted legislation creating a task force to examine the extent of prescription drug abuse among expectant mothers, as well as the costs of caring for babies with Neonatal Abstinence Syndrome, the long-term effects of the syndrome, and prevention strategies.

I was invited to attend a task-force meeting on October 12, 2012, at the Susan B. Anthony Recovery Center, in Broward County. (After touring the facility I learned that each resident mother and child shares an apartment with another mother-child pair. In addition to treatment in the impressive recovery program, women at Susan B. Anthony are taught life skills.)

At the meeting, Dr. William R. Driscoll, associate professor at the University of Florida's Department of Pediatrics Division of Neonatology, spoke about his research regarding NAS babies. I introduced myself to Dr. Driscoll afterwards and asked if he had ever seen a baby who had been exposed to drugs while in the womb but was born asymptomatic (showing no signs of withdrawal). We had a baby on our unit at the time whose mother signed herself out AMA (against medical advice), but left the baby behind. Although she and her baby tested positive for multiple drugs (poly substance abuse), including oxycodone, we were puzzled to find that the baby was not showing evidence of withdrawal.

Dr. Driscoll explained that babies born earlier than thirty-one weeks do not show signs of withdrawal. They do not know why. In this case, the infant showed no signs to alert us, but his mother's behavior certainly did. So, of course, unless the exposure is obvious, as was the case with this infant, the need for intervention will not be evident, and an innocent baby will be sent home, dependent for their every life-sustaining need on a drug-addicted parent. The situation will not come to the attention of authorities until the infant is harmed or killed. While we do not test all babies in Florida for exposure to drugs, perhaps we should. The possibility of universal testing for exposure was discussed in the task-force meeting. Of course, the expense was also noted.

In addition to attending meetings that include legislators and the Attorney General, STOPPNow continued to hold peaceful protests in front of pain clinics. We had no trouble finding pain clinics at which to protest. By 2010, there were over 150 pill mills in Broward County alone, and nearly 1,000 statewide. This was an exponential increase from the mere four pain clinics that existed in Broward in 2007 (an increase that explains the corollary increase in the number of prescription-drug-related deaths and drug-addicted newborns). Those associated with businesses surrounding the pain clinics, local civic organizations, and mothers who knew of the presence of a pain clinic all contacted us with the names of pill mills they wanted shut down.

This moneymaking plan was working out quite well for the clinic owners and for the doctors who worked for them. These are the people who are responsible for the deaths of thousands in our state – including visitors to Florida. The plan was to find doctors who would place greed before respect for a human life. They were able to dispense synthetic heroin (oxycodone) in storefronts to anyone who wanted it. It took years to implement the laws that would begin to affect change. While we were holding protests in 2009, doctors would, for a price, hand out hundreds of pills to their so-called "patients." But in 2010, a law was finally passed to prevent doctors from dispensing narcotics. This did save lives. It did not, however, end the problem. Now, doctors simply write prescriptions, rather than dispense narcotics directly to the patient – and the deaths continue.

Mothers would bring me evidence of the abuse in these prescriptions. One mother gave me a Macy's shopping bag full of copies of prescriptions written and filled for a twenty-seven-year-old male who was not suffering from any illness or injury. The youth was able to walk into a pain clinic and walk out with prescriptions each month. The highest I saw was a prescription for 308 oxycodone (30 mg) and, of course, the usual cocktail of Xanax and Soma. And the pharmacies were filling these high prescriptions. The pharmacy receipts for April 2009 alone for this young man read as follows:

- Post Haste Pharmacy 04/01/09, $585.00

- Affordahealth Dispen (Affordahealth Pain Clinic, same location) 04/09/09, $750.00

- Discount Pharmacy 04/21/09, $960.00

- Affordahealth Dispen 04/24/09, $405.00

All the while, the Board of Medicine (BOM) sat idle as thousands died. Pain clinics could not thrive without a doctor, so the BOM could have saved many lives if they had taken their responsibility seriously. The governor appoints these individuals to their posts. Governors, clean house and choose candidates who will uphold the values stated in their own objectives!

There were many traveling great distances from other states to Florida. Our reputation for having the most beautiful beaches has long been used to promote the South Florida tourist industry. But now, many travel to the Sunshine State because they have learned of the ease with which one can obtain pills.

I received many emails from out of state. Below is an exchange I had with "Luanne" from Massachusetts.

From: Luanne

To: stoppnow@yahoo.com

Date: February 27, 2011

Subject: OxyContin

Good morning. I stumbled on your group's activities while trying to keep up with Florida pill mill news. I live in Massachusetts. Opiate overdose is now the leading cause of death in young people in my state. Nice, huh? Anyway, I am also an RN, and my daughter is an opiate addict, due to illegal OxyContin several years ago that quickly became an addiction, and when she could no longer afford it, she used heroin. She is an IV drug user and has been through hell. She now lives back with us and goes to a methadone clinic every day. Before all this, she was a finance major in college, raised by two parents in a substance-free home. It makes me so mad when people think that it is somehow the parents' fault. It is NOT. This crap is everywhere, and in my daughter's case she was suffering from depression. I think the OxyContin made her feel better –takes away all your troubles. She made a bad decision, for sure. She never used drugs before. Never even drank to excess. So, if this happened to her, you can only imagine what's going on out there.

I go to a support group, Learn to Cope, that has been very good. You should see the parents who come to meetings. It grows every day and recently made a move to a bigger place. The stories are all the same. I will email everyone I can in Florida because the majority of loose Oxy's come from down there. We call it the "Flamingo Express." Rick Scott is missing the boat on this. Also, most of all, I want Purdue Pharma to be closed down, all OxyContin banned, and criminal charges filed against them. We do not need OxyContin for pain control. I know that. It has killed far more people than it has helped.

God bless you ladies for taking time out of your lives to help expose this monster. I have been trying to get more involved, but taking care of my daughter and working doesn't leave much. I love my daughter so much and live in fear for her. She's doing well, but has had some slips. My heart breaks for those who have lost a child to this.

If you have any other suggestions for me to email I will. I emailed Scott and Aronberg and my governor and senators. Also, I am working on a letter to Purdue Pharma. They are right up here in Connecticut. Good luck to you, and keep up the pressure.

Regards,

Luanne

From: stoppnow@yahoo.com

To: Luanne

Date: February 28, 2011

Subject Re: OxyContin

Luanne:

I have been in touch with Director Kerlikowske (National Drug Czar) for some time. I sent his office a copy of your letter. We are going to Tallahassee March 7 and 8. Please write to as many legislators as you can. I offered to go to Washington to try to get something done on a national level. On our website, stoppnow.com, I have included links to media and newspaper articles. This Sunday there was a debate about banning oxycodone. I'll let you know what I hear back. Pray for us.

God bless,

Janet Colbert

From: Luanne

Subject: OxyContin

Date: February 28, 2011

GREAT. You also might want to contact Joanne Peterson. She is the founder of Learn to Cope, a family support group up this way. She knows everything and a lot of people. She has devoted years of her life to this. She's done a LOT. Please look at the website and contact her. So glad to not be alone in this. I have sent and received replies from your Dave Aronberg [in 2011 Dave Aronberg was appointed by Attorney General Pam Bondi, to head the office of Drug Control for Florida. He is now Palm Beach County State Attorney]. He seems OK to me. What's your opinion??

Regards,

Luanne

The following email is from a mother who also found us from the media attention we were getting. She, like all the mothers who have lost their child, will never recover. She used to drive an hour to attend our protests.

From: Kathleen

Subject: Pictures: May 25 Rally

Date: May 25, 2012

After the rally, I went into the consignment shop. The owner said he chases the drugged-up people all the time. He said sometimes they are so high that by the time they reach his door they lose (drop) the scripts they just got. He has a collection of copies. He has turned the originals over to the sheriff's department. He showed them to me. One day one of the doctors wrote a script to the same person, two scripts for oxy 10-mg and one script for 30-mg and one for Xanax 2 mg, all to the same man the same day. The deputy who had been talking to the doctor outside went back in to talk to the store owner. The deputy told the store owner that he asked the doctor why he would prescribe to kids pills that he knows are bad for them. The answer was money, of course. Can you imagine how brazen this doctor is? I hope they get him good when his time comes. While I was there, he chased three guys and called the deputy. He said this goes on daily and he hates it. I wish we had had newspaper coverage on this one.

Kathy

And here is another email:

From: Lisa

Subject: Pain Bee Gone

Date: July 31, 2012

Hi, Ladies:

I'm happy to inform you that Pain Bee Gone is now closed. It was nice driving by and seeing it gone!!! I used to drive up there and preach to whoever would listen. It was sad talking to some of these kids, looking into their eyes and seeing the hurt they have. They don't want to be like this! Something needs to be done to help these kids, even if I make them think about what they're doing. It helps me also! I have learned so much after Heather's passing.

Also, I'm sorry I haven't been out there with everybody. I'm dealing with my son, who's not doing well. This cancer is taking its toll on him. All he wants to do is drugs to forget. I'm fighting this battle of drugs again. These doctors won't listen. They just keep giving him whatever he wants. My heart is broken. I'm so lost

Keep fighting this war. I will be there soon.

Lisa

I say the rosary every day. In addition to my intentions, I always include my request to help the parents who are suffering from the devastating loss of their child (and, in some cases, more than one child). There is the mother who wrote to tell me that she has a part of her basement that she can't clean out. And that once in a while she goes down there and picks up her daughter's things to just smell them. And another mother who was only able to attend the FED UP! Rally in Washington D.C. for one day. She made an appointment to meet with her representative and later told me she didn't cry or throw up or anything. These mothers have been thrown into this role without asking – suffering their loss and wanting to prevent it from happening to another.

CHAPTER FOUR

The Cause

In Chapter Three, you read about some of the effects of this prescription-pill epidemic. Now, let me introduce you to the cause – greed.

For instance, Dr. Selwyn Carrington, a successful South Florida endocrinologist, found prescribing painkillers as a way to supplement his income. However, Dr. Carrington was caught and charged.

The FBI Miami Division U.S. Attorney's Office March 25, 2011: Doctor Charged with Conspiring to Distribute Controlled Substances.

The criminal complaint charges the defendant, Dr. Carrington, with conspiring to dispense and distribute and to cause the dispensing and distribution of controlled substances through medical clinics in Hallandale and West Palm Beach, Florida ... If convicted, Dr. Carrington faces a maximum statutory sentence of twenty years. Selwyn is a licensed physician in the State of Florida.

According to court documents, the investigation revealed that Dr. Carrington did not treat or evaluate any clients at the clinics, and he was not at the clinics during normal business hours. Further, the investigation revealed that in exchange for $5,000 per month, Dr. Carrington only went to the clinics approximately once per week to sign progress notes for patients who had been previously seen by the ARNPs (Advanced Registered

Nurse Practitioners) and to pre-sign blank prescriptions so the ARNPs and other employees, who have no medical licenses, could illegally prescribe controlled substances to their clients. According to the charging documents, Percocet, oxycodone, and Xanax were all illegally prescribed in this manner.

An analysis of the payments made by Florida Medicaid for the time period from March 2005 through January 2011 indicated that over 300,000 pills containing controlled substances were dispensed to Primary Care Practitioners' clients due to the prescriptions pre-signed by Dr. Carrington. The Florida Medicaid Program paid for these pills.

Doctor Carrington had privileges at the very hospital I worked for. And the hospital did not like what I was doing by calling attention to the pill mills? There are many honest, hard-working people who arise early in the morning, work all week, and do not make $60,000 a year. This is the amount he was making from pre-signing illegal prescriptions – in addition to his endocrinology practice. But he probably made more, as there is no mention of the pills that were paid for in cash.

In this case, there was some measure of justice.

STATE OF FLORIDA BOARD OF MEDICINE

Department of Health, Petitioner vs. Selwyn Carrington, M.D., Respondent

This Cause came before the Board of Medicine on November 30, 2012, for consideration of the Administrative Complaint. The facts are not in dispute. Upon consideration, it is ordered: The violations set forth warrant disciplinary action by the Board.

THEREFORE, IT IS HEREBY ORDERED AND ADJUDGED:

Respondent's license to practice medicine in the State of Florida is hereby REVOKED.

Unfortunately, the removal of a medical license from a doctor who is not acting in the best interest of a patient is not the norm. Many doctors practice for years who should have been stopped in order to save lives. For instance, let me share the case of Dr. Cynthia Cadet, whose medical licensure status I have monitored for years.

Dr. Cadet made $1.3 million dollars in the fifteen months she worked at the pill mill known as American Pain Clinic, located at 5801 N. Federal Highway, Boca Raton, Florida, and thereafter, at 1200 North Dixie Highway, Lake Worth, Florida. The pain clinics involved were owned by the George brothers. (There is more to come about the George brothers.) Although Dr. Cadet was charged in connection with six deaths, she, along with one other doctor, Dr. Joseph Castronuovo, were the only two doctors in the practice who did not accept a plea bargain on the charge of money laundering that was offered to them – which had been taken by the other medical staff at the pain clinic at the time of their arrest. The jury convicted both Cadet and Castronuovo, but only of money laundering.

The violations took place in 2009. Dr. Cynthia Cadet voluntarily relinquished her license to practice medicine on July 29, 2016. This lag time makes me ask how many deaths could have been prevented if the Board of Medicine (BOM) removed licensure in a timely manner?

Below is the hearing of U.S. Department of Justice and DEA for removal of Dr. Cynthia Cadet's DEA license.

U.S. Department of Justice Drug Enforcement Administration

OFFICE OF DIVERSION CONTROL

April 7, 2011, Department of Justice

I order that DEA Certificate of Registration, issued to Cynthia M. Cadet, M.D., be and it hereby is revoked. This Order is effective immediately. Dated: March 31, 2011 Michele M. Leonhart, Administrator.

At the hearing, the Government presented the testimony of three witnesses, [two of whom are] DEA Miami Field Division Group Supervisor (GS) Susan Langston [and] DEA Specialist Agent (SA) Michael Burt. GS Langston testified that the investigation of the American Pain Clinic had its origins on November 30, 2009, during a routine inspection that she and a subordinate diversion investigator conducted at a pharmacy doing business under the name Boca Drugs, and located a few blocks away from one of the former locations of American Pain. According to Langston, an examination of the prescriptions seized from Boca Drugs revealed that the majority of those prescriptions were for oxycodone and alprazolam authorized over the signature of physicians associated with American Pain... from November 2, 2009, through November 25, 2009, 151 controlled-substance prescriptions issued over the Respondent's signature [Cynthia Cadet] to seventy-eight patients, only seven of whom resided in Florida. The remainder of the patients had listed addresses in Kentucky, Tennessee, Ohio, Georgia, West Virginia, Indiana, and Missouri.

GS Langston also testified that, on March 3, 2010, a criminal search warrant was executed on the American Pain Clinic...According to Langston, the items seized from American Pain included a sign that had been posted in what she believes to have served as the urinalysis waiting room: *Attention Patients: Due to increased fraudulent prescriptions, it's best if you fill your medication in Florida or your regular pharmacy. Don't go to a pharmacy in Ohio when you live in Kentucky and had the scripts written in Florida. The police will confiscate your scripts and hold them while they investigate. This will take up to six months. So only fill your meds in Florida or a pharmacy that you have been using for at least three months.* The respondent prescribed and dispensed inordinate amounts of controlled substances, primarily oxycodone. It was established that Cynthia Cadet knew or should have known that the prescriptions were not dispensed for a legitimate medical purpose.

Testimony was also given by S.A. Burt.

Based on these surveillance efforts, S.A. Burt testified concerning various activities he observed occurring outside the Boca and Lake Worth clinic locations, which were open to the public from 8:00 a.m. to 5:00 p.m. At the Boca location, Burt stated that on any given day, beginning at 7:00 a.m., automobiles could be seen pulling into the parking lot and approximately twenty to thirty people were routinely lined up outside of the clinic waiting to gain admittance. Additionally, there was a steady stream of automobile and foot traffic in and out of the clinic throughout the day. Burt testified that in his estimation, approximately eighty to ninety percent of the automobiles had out-of-state tags, predominantly from Kentucky, Ohio, West Virginia, and Tennessee.

The next witness to testify at the hearing was a doctor who was an expert witness called in to review the files, Dr. Kennedy.

Kennedy observed that comparing the patient charts, basically it's the same. The patients are given high-dose oxycodone and two different strengths. The Roxicodone 15mg is twice a day (60 pills). Roxicodone 30mg is given six times a day (180 pills) in one case and eight times a day in another (240 pills). Xanax 2 mg.

Dr. Kennedy, in the reviewed charts, included the relatively young age of the Respondent's chronic pain patients, incomplete history information provided by the patients, periodically significant gaps between office visits, referrals from friends, relatives, or advertising, but not other physicians. He also referenced the fact that a relatively high number of patients were traveling significant distances to American Pain for pain treatment, although no physician employed at that facility had any specialized training in pain management.

Dr. Kennedy concluded his report regarding the Respondent's prescribing practices with the following summary:

The Respondent was not engaged in the practice of medicine. Rather, she was engaged in an efficient, assembly line business...She prescribed controlled substances so that patients would return to the office on a regular basis. The Respondent's routine and excessive prescription of multiple controlled substances (oxycodone and Xanax) and lack of arriving at a valid medical diagnosis and treatment most likely caused harm to the patients she saw. Drug diversion most likely caused a "mushroom" effect of drug abuse, drug addiction, drug overdoses, serious bodily injury, and death in those communities spread over several different states. The Respondent's continued ability to prescribe controlled substances will only perpetuate the suffering and be a threat to the public.

Why doesn't the BOM revoke a medical license in a timely manner? To answer that question one only has to look to the Florida Medical Board Regulations.

To begin with, there is also no scientific evidence that supports the use of the opiate in treating chronic pain. And some of the regulations look as though they were written for the Board by the drug companies. The regulations are in serious need of being updated. Since 2010, it has been unlawful for a physician to dispense Schedule II, III, or IV drugs from their office. But the Board's regulations should not create a situation in which those breaking the law need have no fear of disciplinary action for dispensing.

Consider the regulations for yourself:

Florida Medical Board Regulations

64B8-9.013 Standards for the Use of Controlled Substances for the Treatment of Pain.

(b) Inadequate pain control may result from physicians' lack of knowledge about pain management or an inadequate understanding of addiction. Fears of investigation or sanction by federal, state, and local regulatory agencies may also result in inappropriate or inadequate treatment of chronic pain patients. Physicians should not fear disciplinary action from the Board of other state regulatory or enforcement agencies for prescribing, dispensing, or administering controlled substances including opioid analgesics, for a legitimate medical purpose and that is supported by appropriate documentation establishing a valid medical need and treatment plan.

(c) Physicians should recognize that tolerance and physical dependence are normal consequences of sustained use of opioid analgesics and are not synonymous with addiction.

(f) Each case of prescribing for pain will be evaluated on an individual basis. The Board will not take disciplinary action against a physician for failing to adhere strictly to the provisions of these standards, if good cause is shown for such deviation.

(g) The Board will judge the validity of prescribing based on the physician's treatment of the patient and on available documentation, rather than on the quantity and chronicity of prescribing.

If these are the standards, why even have them?

Below is the status of Dr. Cynthia Cadet's medical license being voluntarily revoked. A complaint must be filed and reviewed by the Medical Quality Assurance (MQA); they refer recommendations to the BOM or dismiss the complaint.

Found on the Department of Health License Verification site:

>Controlled Substance Prescriber: No (the DEA revoked her DEA license)

>Discipline on File: No

>Public Complaint: Yes

>Alerts: Voluntary Relinquishment of License filed on 06/22/2016

Dr. Cynthia Cadet relinquished her license to practice medicine five years after the DEA revoked her license. This voluntary relinquishment of license came three years after a federal jury cleared her of six overdose deaths, but convicted her of money laundering. The overprescribing practices and jury verdict of guilty of money laundering are listed below in a condensed version:

State of Florida Department of Health Petitioner V Cynthia Cadet, M.D.

Case No: 2010-08048

During the course of treatment, Respondent prescribed combinations of controlled substances to JA, including Roxicodone and Xanax. The dosages began with Roxicodone 30 mg #210, Roxicodone 15mg #60 and Xanax 2 mg #30. Over the course of treatment, Respondent increased the quantities of the prescriptions Roxicodone 30 mg #240, Roxicodone 15mg #90, and Xanax 2mg # 75 with no written justification.

On or about and between November 2, 2009, and February 23, 2010, Patient RA presented to Respondent for treatment. Respondent prescribed

Roxicodone 30 mg # 240, Roxicodone 15 mg # 60 increasing to # 90 and Xanax 2 mg # 30.

State of Florida Department of Health Petitioner V Cynthia Maley Cadet, M.D.

Case no: 2011-13720

By a Second Superseding Indictment filed on July 19, 2012, in Case No. 10-801149-CR, in the United States District Court for the Southern District of Florida, Respondent was charged with multiple counts of violations of the United States Code related to her practice at American Pain Clinic. It is further alleged that the specified unlawful activity is the distribution, dispensing, and possession with intent to distribute and dispense, oxycodone, a Schedule II narcotic controlled substance, outside the scope of professional practice and not for a legitimate medical purpose. Respondent was convicted by jury verdict of violating Count 13. The Offenses charged in Count 13 are otherwise commonly referred to as "money laundering."

There is another case, Case No: 2009-15100, that spans the terms of two Florida State Surgeons General. The first was signed on December, 22, 2011, by State Surgeon General H. Frank Farmer, Jr., M.D. The second, an Amended Administrative Complaint of Case No: 2009-15100, was signed by State Surgeon General John H. Armstrong, M.D., on June 29, 2015. Both documents describe inappropriately and excessively prescribing controlled substances in potentially lethal combinations and doses, to Patient TG, without medical justification.

Therein lies the problem. Cynthia Cadet voluntary relinquished her license to practice medicine June 2016. She had been prescribing excessive amounts of the opiate along with other addictive drugs since 2009. This is shameful, Board of Medicine. We are still, to this day, trying to have laws enacted that will stop the carnage.

CHAPTER FIVE

Politicians

The sting of so many parents suffering the same loss was exacerbated by the lack of political interest in generating a solution, which has brought us to where we are today: more deaths. I wrote letters to many politicians. I naively thought once they realized what was happening in our state and in our country, they would take measures needed to end this tragedy. The first letter was written in July 2010. (Unbeknownst to me at the time, I would continue to follow the George brothers and the death of a young man named Joseph Bartolucci that meant so little to them, but which troubled me so much. More about Joseph Bartolucci's death and the George brothers will follow later. But they did get their Lamborghini taken, eventually, and I had a front row seat for those proceedings.)

Attorney General of Florida Bill McCollum
State of Florida the Capital Pl – 01
Tallahassee, FL 32399-1050

July 7, 2010

Dear Attorney General Bill McCollum:

I am a neonatal intensive care RN. I am disturbed over the suffering of infants born into the horrible world of drug abuse and withdrawal. The number of babies being born addicted to drugs has drastically and alarmingly increased.

We have not only observed the increase in the amount of cases but also the severity of symptoms. Please also consider the lives these children have once they leave our unit. Many of the infants are on HRS hold and spend their lives in the foster care system. If the lives of these babies are not considered valuable, perhaps the cost to the state as a result might be important.

It has come to my attention that when Governor Crist was attorney general in 2004, he hailed the indictment of a physician named Solis. A federal grand jury in Miami unsealed a fifteen-count indictment against Solis—one count conspiring to defraud the federal government, one count conspiring to distribute controlled substances, and thirteen counts distributing controlled substances. In the article, he referred to this physician as "a drug dealer in a white coat." You are aware that M.D.s do not always honor the Hippocratic Oath they take.

There are over 100 pain clinics in Broward County alone. I am including a medical examiner's report of deaths in Broward County. These deaths are all due to prescription drug overdoses.

2005 - 21 deaths

2006 - 45 deaths

2007 - 65 deaths

2008 - 92 deaths

2009 - 82 deaths

(Partial year 05/10) 43 deaths.

As staggering as these figures are, they don't include all of the deaths as a result of the pain clinics. A letter included from my friend of many years when our children were babies themselves describes her son's death. Although he was entwined in this pain clinic maelstrom, his death was the result of a motor vehicle hit and run. The numbers above are only the tip of the iceberg. And this is only one county in Florida.

I am also including an article quoting a pain clinic owner. This article is from the *Palm Beach Post*, by Michael LaForgia. The article describes the death of a twenty-four-year old due to an overdose for drugs received from East Coast Pain Clinic.

> "Whatever I'm worth, I've earned it," said George, 29, who has no medical background. "Whether it's a thousand dollars, a million, or ten million dollars."
>
> Besides East Coast Pain Clinic, George runs clinics in Hallandale Beach and Hollywood.
>
> "We take every precaution and every measure to assure this doesn't happen," Jeffery George said, Friday, of fatal overdoses. "Unfortunately, the clinic and the doctor can't control a patient if they go home and do something stupid."
>
> "I bought my Lamborghini four years ago," he added. "If I wreck it, am I going to hold the Lamborghini dealership responsible?"

This businessman/criminal places no value on a human life. There are nineteen pages of deaths from the medical examiner's office due to drug overdoses of prescribed medications that are from pain clinics. Mr. George must have been too busy counting his money when Toyota executives were called to testify regarding deaths due to Toyota's sudden acceleration. Please help us to take his Lamborghini and his flippant attitude away.

I do not understand why a blind eye is turned to these pain clinics being allowed to operate. They are drug dealers with a license to kill. If they are not operating outside the law, then the law needs to change.

Please google "OxyContin Express" and watch what our politicians have allowed South Florida to become.

Sincerely,

Janet Colbert RNC
and Michael

I did not receive an answer to this letter. My next request was inviting the Attorney General to our rally.

Attorney General of Florida Bill McCollum
State of Florida the Capital Pl – 01
Tallahassee, FL 32399-1050

August 9, 2010

Dear Attorney General Bill McCollum:

I invite you to join us for a peaceful demonstration to close the pain clinics on Tuesday, August 24, 2010, at 9:00 a.m., at the Pain Relief clinic located at 3088 Griffin Road, Fort Lauderdale, Florida, 33312.

You should be ashamed to hold/or run for office in our state if you have no intention of closing the pain clinics. I do not like living in a community that you have permitted to become the OxyContin capital. We would welcome your support at our rally. And let's together do whatever is necessary to change the laws that are allowing legalized drug dealers to flourish.

Sincerely,
STOPPNow
Janet Colbert, RNC, BSN, IBCLC
and Michael

This is not the best way to go about trying to make change. But even though this was early on in this fight my passion and frustration were showing. When we started our organization, there were over 150 pill mills in just Broward County (more than McDonalds). I just could not understand why it was and still is so hard to get those who are in office to allow this to continue. As you may have guessed, he was not at our rally, nor did I get an answer.

Attorney General of Florida Bill McCollum

State of Florida the Capital Pl – 01
Tallahassee, FL 32399-1050

August 31, 2010

Dear Attorney General Bill McCollum:

I do not know what your future aspirations are for political office but if you want a vote in South Florida you will file a bill to close the pain clinics.

Our first rally was very successful. This is a subject that is volatile in South Florida. It has affected many families. I've written to you before regarding the drug addicted babies born in our community, and they are still coming. If your answer is to continue to ignore this, then we do not need you representing us.

Sincerely,
Janet Colbert RNC
and Michael

Again, no response.

Governor Charles Crist
The Capitol 400 S. Monroe Street
Tallahassee, Florida 32399-0001

Cc:

Broward County Commissioner
John E. Rodstrom, Jr
Broward County Governmental Center Room 416
115 S. Andrews Avenue
Ft. Lauderdale, Florida 33301

Commissioner Bobbie H Grace
100 N. Dania Beach Blvd
Dania Beach, Florida 33004

June 16, 2010

Dear Governor:

We are writing to you as concerned citizens of Broward County. I work in a neonatal intensive care unit in one of Broward County's hospitals. The number of our babies being born addicted to drugs has drastically and alarmingly increased. We administer morphine every three hours and sometimes a necessary second drug to these babies trying to help them through the drug withdrawal torment they are born with. We have not only observed the increase in the amount of cases, but also the severity of symptoms. It is pitiful to hold a baby who is screaming and trembling and despite his hunger has the inability to control his oral musculature enough to enable him to suck a bottle. The enormity of the problem is not isolated to our unit I'm sure, but rather dispersed throughout our county.

We are hoping you will help us with stopping the supply portion of the supply-and-demand equation of drug addiction. There are over 150 pain clinics in Broward County. Young, childbearing-aged women are filling prescriptions, legally. Medical doctors are issuing these prescriptions, and our pharmacies are filling them. Never mind closing the borders from Mexico, we have a problem right here in our own county. Many of these pain clinics advertise on-site dispensing. These M.D./drug dealers are not arrested, and they are not losing their licenses. They may not be breaking any laws but they are trafficking drugs. We need to change the law. We must close these pain clinics; they are not legitimate businesses.

We will be happy to meet with you and if able present our data at a county commissioners meeting. Please view www.oxycontinexpress.com (tab Vanguard). Broward County has earned a reputation that we must change.

Please help us help the babies not yet born into this hellish addiction.

Sincerely,
Janet Colbert RNC
and Michael

STOPPNow

———

Governor Charles Crist
The Capital 400 S. Monroe Street
Tallahassee, Florida 32399-0001

July11, 2010

Dear Governor Crist:

This is my second letter to you regarding my concern relating to the pain clinics that are allowed to legally operate in South Florida. Three of us have formed an organization named STOPPNow (Stop the Organized Pill Pushers Now). We three have written individual letters all with a story to share. We do plan to demonstrate in front of these pain clinics to draw attention in order to rectify this wrong.

I am a neonatal intensive care RN. Not only am I disturbed over the suffering of these neonates being born into a horrible world of drug abuse and withdrawal, but also please consider as I do the lives these children have once they leave our unit. They are on HRS hold and spend their lives in the foster care system. If the lives of these children are not being considered valuable, then perhaps the cost that the state will have to incur as a result might be important.

It has come to my attention, Governor Crist, that as attorney general for our state in 2004 you hailed the indictment of a physician named Solis. You are aware that M.D.s do not always honor the Hippocratic Oath they take: I will do no harm.

There are over 100 pain clinics in Broward County alone. I received a report from the Broward County Medical Examiner's Office. It contains nineteen pages of deaths due to oxycodone. From 2005 until present, the deaths have increased 433 percent. There is a direct correlation between the increased number of deaths and the multiplication of pain clinics populating Broward County. Bear in mind that every pill that caused these deaths was prescribed by a physician.

An article in the *Palm Beach Post*, written by staff writer Michael LaForgia, on June 30, 2010, is titled: "Oxycodone Overdose Deaths Jump 26% Statewide." This is a statewide problem due to the law, or lack thereof, in Florida.

You strive for success and growth in your political career. Your service as governor for the state of Florida must include the closure of the pain clinics. Take their license to operate away. What more do you need?

I am also including an article quoting a pain clinic owner.

I do not understand why the elected officials are endorsing the operation of these pain clinics. After all, they are licensed to operate. They are drug dealers with a license to kill. If they are not operating outside the law, then the law needs to be changed.

Please google "OxyContin Express" and watch what the politicians have allowed South Florida to become.

Janet Colbert RNC
and Michael

I did receive a letter back from the Office of the Governor dated July 13, 2010. Below is my response to the letter I received from the Governor's office.

Mr. Andrew J. Benard
Chief of Staff Governor Charles Crist
Florida Office of Drug control

July 23, 2010

Dear Mr. Benard:

We have organized a group since my first letter to Governor Crist. We sent letters to Governor Crist and other representatives a few days before I received your letter in response to my letter to Governor Crist. I am including in this correspondence a letter that was written to a judge on behalf of a young girl who was present when this woman's son died from a drug overdose. As you can see there is no malice in this mother's plea to help the girl avoid prosecution rather than condemn her. Too many families are suffering. The young man died from oxycodone, Xanax, and soma, which he received from a pain clinic…

This tragedy took place before the Good Samaritan law was passed in Florida. The Good Samaritan law encourages those at the scene of an overdose to call for help without any threat of reprisal. The young girl mentioned above did try to do the right thing. She awakened her mother, who administered CPR while waiting for emergency services to arrive. All efforts to save the young man's life were unsuccessful. Drug paraphernalia was found at the scene, and the seventeen-year-old girl was arrested. Meanwhile, the doctor and pain clinic owner went to the bank to make their deposit for the day.

….Perhaps you and Governor Crist should visit our neonatal intensive care unit and hold a baby who is born withdrawing from drugs.

We are aware of House Bill 2272; however, this falls short of our expectations. When people – a lot of people – are packing their cars and traveling on airplanes from other states to buy drugs in Florida, something is wrong. I'd like to address matters in your letter that suggest to me that you are not aware, perhaps, of the enormity of the problem. You write, "The illegal diversion of prescription drugs – scheduled drugs prescribed by physicians, but then diverted from their intended use to be abused or illegally sold – also increases crime and human suffering." This is only a small part of the problem. In the big picture, these physicians are not physicians. They may have a license to practice, but that is your fault. There are ten pages of advertisements for pain clinics in a magazine titled the *New Times*, where they blatantly advertise for drug users to frequent their establishment. A few examples:

No Florida ID necessary

Dr. Bentley is gone. (Maybe you should interview Dr. Bentley)

In-house dispensing

We see walk-in new patients at any time with no long lectures.

They advertise on the same page with ads for penis enlargement and escort services. Do not write to me as if these are legitimate doctors. I work with real doctors. The neonatologists I work with constantly study research to improve quality of life and strive to save lives.

Many people are interested in what we have started. We are going to have a rally in front of a pain clinic, and we will not stop until they are all closed. You can be seen as trying to do something or as endorsing them.

We will be happy to meet with the legislative branch when they are in session and plead our case to change the necessary laws to stop the operation of legalized drug dealing. Will you help us to change the law?

In other states, pain sufferers can obtain relief from their own doctors (oncologists, orthopedic surgeons). These pain clinics are just a farce and never should have received a license to operate.

Sincerely,
Janet Colbert
and Michael

Governor Charles Christ
The Capitol
400 S. Monroe Street
Tallahassee, Florida 32399-0001

August 9, 2010

Dear Governor Crist:

I invite you to join us for a peaceful demonstration to close the pain clinics on Tuesday, August 24, 2010, at 9:00 a.m. at the Pain Relief Center located at 3088 Griffin Road, Fort Lauderdale, Florida 33312.

You should be ashamed to hold or run for office in our state if you have no intention of closing the pain clinics. I do not like living in a community that you have permitted to become the OxyContin capital. We would welcome your support at our rally. And let's, together, do whatever is necessary to change the laws that are allowing legalized drug dealers to flourish.

Sincerely,
STOPPNow
Janet Colbert RNC, BSN, IBCLC
and Michael

Governor Charles Crist
The Capitol
400 S. Monroe Street
Tallahassee, Florida 32399-0001

August 29, 2010

Dear Governor Crist:

Our organization is growing. Our first rally was very successful. In 2007 there were four pain clinics in Broward County. Now, there are 150. We have a website, stoppnow.com, and people are paying attention.

You are not going to win the South Florida vote unless you take a stand to close the pain clinics. We need you to file a bill to close the pain clinics. We will help support the effective change needed.

If this matter is not important to you then you have no business asking for our vote. I will be sending letters to Marco Rubio and Kendrick Meeks. The next senator should be the man who truly represents the people. Look how far Senator Marco Rubio has come. He has done nothing to stop the deaths.

Our next rally will be held Monday, September 20, 2010. I again invite you to attend.

Sincerely,
Janet Colbert
and Michael

These letters were written when Charlie Crist was the governor of Florida and still a Republican. He did lose the election for governor to Governor Rick Scott. Rick Scott was against passage of the Prescription Drug Monitoring Program (PDMP), the database that tracks prescriptions written by doctors for narcotics and the patients who fill them. The opposition caused a delay in its passage. It did go into effect October, 2011. STOPPNow did make a trip to Tallahassee. We met with Governor Rick Scott's office. We also met with then-President of the Florida Senate, Mike Haridopolos. He promised us that the PDMP would pass. I hope he runs for the U.S. Senate. He and his wife Stephanie are wonderful people. On this same trip to Tallahassee, we met with representatives of the Attorney General's office. The meeting was arranged by Dave Aronberg, appointed by Attorney General Pam Bondi to the position of Head of Florida's Drug Task Force.

As we went around the table and introduced ourselves, one of the gentlemen present at the table was Andrew Benard. His face turned beet red when I reminded him of the letter I sent to him July of 2010, while he was Chief of Staff Florida Office of Drug Control under then-Governor Charlie Crist.

We spent a good part of that afternoon conversing with the Attorney General's team. I have talked on many occasions with Andrew Benard since then. It was nice to get to know them and put a face to those with whom we were conversing through letters and emails. Andrew Benard is still with the Attorney General's office. I truly believe he is one of the good guys and shares my frustration that after so many years we are still not able to stop the deaths.

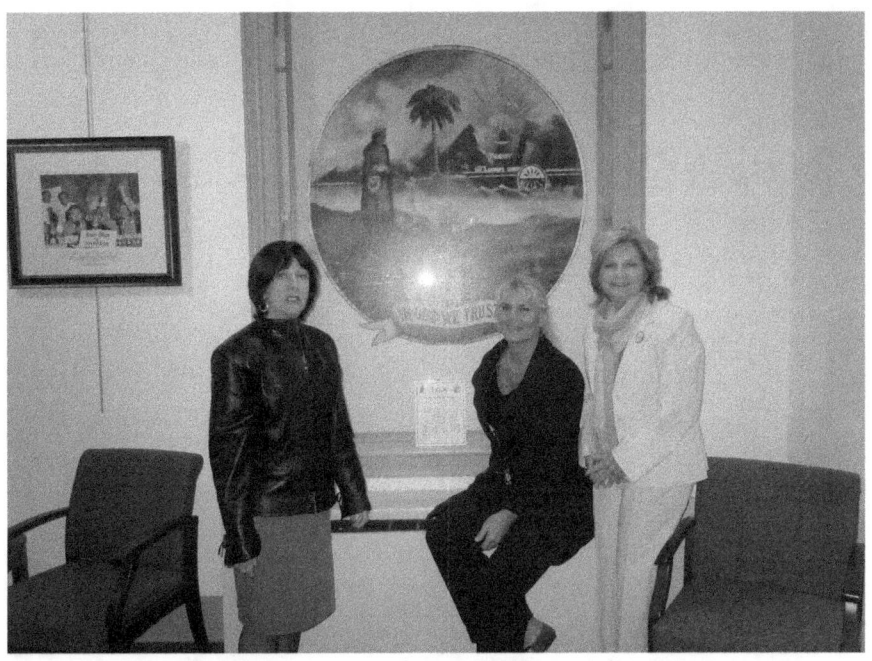
Janet, Joy, and Renee in Tallahassee Florida

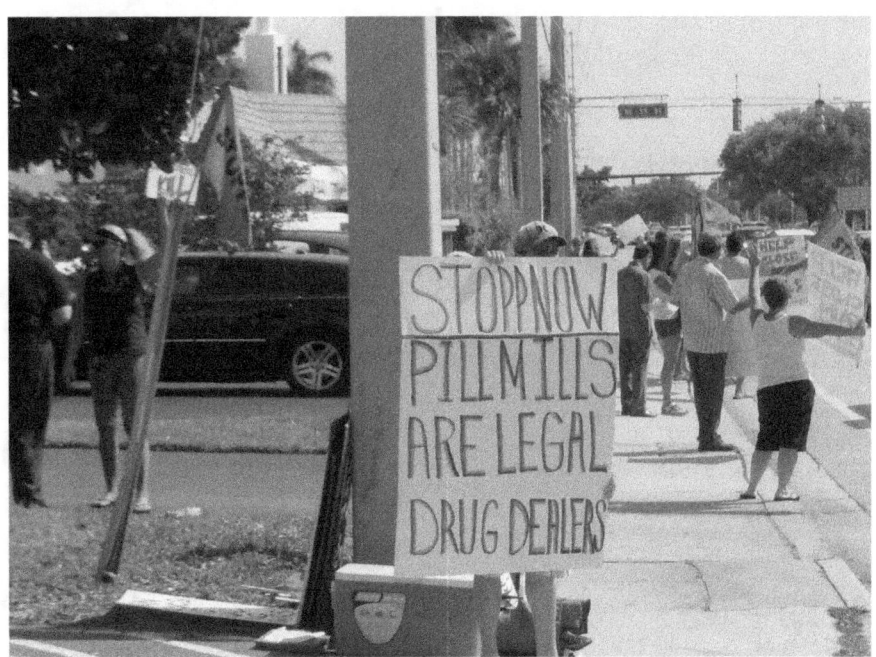
Peaceful protest.

CHAPTER SIX

Senator Eleanor Sobel

On January 29, 2014, Maureen and I were able to make an appointment for a conference call with Senator Sobel. I asked Senator Sobel if she had a chance to read the information we had sent for her to review and needed her support for. Senator Sobel said that her aide, Jeremy, had given her nothing and we should explain. I began telling her that we would like the PDMP to be made mandatory for usage by the doctors prior to writing a prescription for narcotics.

She immediately answered, "We don't have doctors writing scripts for 200 pills."

I told her I have seen scripts for more than 300 pills. We told her the subpoena had been placed back in Florida Senate Bill SPB 7014. (There are those who oppose the PDMP and are trying to dismantle it. The subpoena would require law enforcement to obtain a subpoena before checking the PDMP).

Senator Sobel asked Jeremy to check and found we were correct. Her plans are to vote against the bill due to the subpoena, and we agree with her on that point. STOPPNow takes the position that law enforcement is the only agency trying to eradicate this epidemic, and why would there be a push to restrict their efforts? We were told at the initiation of the PDMP that every year we could work towards strengthening it. I believe the subpoena is an effort to suppress any improvements to the database. Rather, valuable time is now being spent just to be able to keep it.

Senator Sobel stated that mandating the usage of the PDMP only creates more paperwork for the doctors, and that there had already been an effort in the past to make it mandatory, and why would we throw that in again. I told her we were aware that Senator Fasano had written the PDMP with inclusion of the mandatory component for physicians to use, and Representative Ronald Renuart amended the bill to remove the mandate.

I also asked that she support the interstate exchange, as Florida almost wiped out an entire generation in Clay County, Kentucky, where there are only two industries: coal mining and selling drugs. Maureen told Senator Sobel that she had spoken to Rebecca Poston, Program Director of the PDMP, known as Electronic-Florida Online Reporting of Controlled Substance Evaluation Program (E-FORCSE), and learned that currently twenty-five percent of the prescriptions for drugs are going to Alabama.

Senator Sobel's response was, "I don't care about Alabama or Kentucky. I only care about Florida."

I was incensed by her response. Not only should she not be a state senator, who, one would think, should be held in esteem. But what a poor excuse for a human being. I composed myself enough to say that it is Florida doctors that are writing the prescriptions. Twenty-one states at the time were participating in the interstate exchange, and Florida should be one of them. Her response was that it would never fly, that it was not a good idea for names to be given out to other states.

Maureen brought up the fact that the BOM and Department of Health (DOH), as shown on E-FORCSE records, had only utilized the PDMP six times in one year. Maureen also brought up the fact that doctors are still overprescribing, and that this never would have become such a problem if the BOM had taken away licensure of high-prescribing doctors: No doctor equals no pain clinic. Maureen further explained that we have been at BOM meetings. The BOM only gives doctors a slap on the wrist, and they go right back to the pill mill.

Senator Sobel said that we should call the newspapers. I said that we have been in the newspapers many times; that we need legislation to put an end to this, and this was why we were coming to her. I told her of the doctors making half-a-million dollars a year and who, when brought before the BOM, are only fined $15,000. This is not a deterrent for them to stop, and worst of all they leave the BOM meeting with a clear license to practice.

Maureen brought up clinic owner Vincent Coangello. At the time of his arrest, he was making $150,000 a day. His clinic was raided by the DEA. (Again, law enforcement is the only agency we have trying to stop this.) Yet all of the doctors who worked for that pill mill maintained their licenses to practice and have never been brought to justice for their part.

Senator Sobel's response was, "$150,000 a day. That's a lot of money."

This conversation was very disheartening. It was clear we were speaking to someone who just didn't care. Somewhere in the conversation, Senator Sobel said she didn't know why we were trying to explode the whole PDMP. She said currently she would vote against the bill. She listed the inclusion of law enforcement's need for a subpoena as the reason. "If the bill is going to be voted down, because most of the committee is in agreement with me, why would we want to tack this on anyway?" she asked.

Senator Sobel makes a good point, but why would it have to be tacked on to that bill? I assured her our efforts were to strengthen the PDMP and not for it to be in jeopardy. We are trying to save lives. Senator Sobel's response: "I save lives every day."

When Senator Sobel spoke of the mandatory component and the extra work for doctors she said about fifty percent of doctors don't have electronic equipment. Maureen told her there is a law that requires the doctors to have the electronic system in place. Senator Sobel's response was, "Yeah, but that's not in effect yet."

When I called her on the fifty percent, she said she didn't know exactly how many doctors. I understand why this has gone on for so long in Florida after speaking to the Senator. She seemed clueless and not willing to change anything. Meanwhile, we had no intention of giving up.

CHAPTER SEVEN

The Taking Down of Joel Shumrak

We continued to hold peaceful protests in front of pain clinics to draw much needed attention. The deaths continued to rise. One mother, who had lost her daughter as a result of that pain clinic, used to wear her daughter's ashes around her neck as she walked up and down the sidewalk in front of the clinic with us. The daughter's boyfriend was also a fatality of this pain clinic. The two died within weeks of each other. The owner of the Pain Center of Broward used to stand outside alongside his security guard, Glock on hip, watching us. He'd sometimes call the police, but we were allowed to be there, and we protested in front of Joel Shumrak's clinic in Fort Lauderdale numerous times over many years.

Then, in June 2014, something I never thought would occur happened. One of the Broward County Commissioners, Chip LaMarca – who has been out in front of pain clinics, Shumrak's included, protesting with us on more than one occasion – contacted me to tell me something big was going on at the Pain Center of Broward. I was on the computer when this email came in:

> From: LaMarca, Chip
> To: Stoppnow@yahoo.com
> Date: June 3, 2014

> I just drove by the pill mill on North Federal in Fort Lauderdale saw a wonderful sight of Fort Lauderdale PD, Department of Health, and what appeared to be federal agents. Hopefully they can shut this place down for good.

Best Regards,
Chip LaMarca,
Broward County Commissioner

I knew exactly which pill mill he was referring to. Maureen lives close to Joel Shumrak, Pain Center of Broward. I quickly called her.

From: Stoppnow@yahoo.com
Subject: Re:
To: LaMarca, Chip

Thanks, Chip. Maureen lives close. She's on her way over.

Janet

The raid involved our DEA working in conjunction with Kentucky DEA. Law enforcement in Kentucky was well aware that pill bottles left behind the scene of an overdose death in Kentucky had come all the way from Broward County, Florida. So, although Tallahassee, Florida, legislators don't care about people dying in Kentucky or Alabama, law enforcement and the DEA do. Kentucky had had enough of Joel Shumrak and the Pain Center of Broward. Joel Shumrak was extradited to Kentucky.

This was the second raid that took place at this pain clinic. Carmel Cafiero, who is employed by WSVN, a local news station, tells the story, below. We have seen and spoken to her many times, and she is an avid reporter (like a little bull dog). She gets right in their faces. She would often be seen on the evening news running through parking lots after the owners or doctors of a pill mill. This particular incident took place in 2012. It would still be another two years before the clinic was raided and closed for good.

Carmel Cafiero: "Good morning. Are you Mr. Shumrak?"

Joel Shumrak: "No."

Carmel Cafiero: "You're not?"

It was Shumrak. Carmel Cafiero was questioning Shumrak about Dr. Leonard Haimes, who worked for Shumrak until the doctor's license was suspended. The state accused him of prescribing more than 10,000 highly addictive oxycodone and other pain pills to five patients.

>Cafiero: "I'd like to talk with you about Dr. Haimes and the suspension."

>Shumrak: "I can't talk about Dr. Haimes."

>Cafiero: "Why not? This is your clinic." [This is the bulldog I mentioned earlier].

When this raid took place, the doctor was arrested. As files were being removed and the doctor escorted out in handcuffs, Joel Shumrak stated that he would reopen by Thursday. Sure enough, the pill mill was open for business before the end of the week. They advertise for doctors on Craig's List and have no trouble filling the position. Greed.

I have many stories on things observed while out on that sidewalk protesting. At one protest, while I was in the parking lot next door with a mother and a detective, I noticed the Ft. Lauderdale police car take off from where he was perched and fly into the parking lot of the pill mill.

I ran over. The mothers began telling me that they all heard this loud bang; they thought it was a gunshot. They told of the young man who had come out of the pain clinic and started to drive away. He hit something and staggered out of his car to see what he had hit. It was one of those large dumpsters.

The security guard told the policeman that the pill mill customer did not hit anything. There were five mothers there who witnessed it and stated he could hardly stand up and was staggering as he made his way to the back of the car to see what he had run into.

The officer's response to us was that the guard said he didn't hit anything. This clinic's address is 5459 North Federal Highway. Federal Highway (US1) is a very busy, six-lane highway. I said to the policemen, "Surely, you are not going to let him drive his car out of this parking lot and onto this street, are you?"

His response was that he, the policeman, staggers sometimes when he walks. And, sure enough, he let the client, who could hardly stand up, drive away onto the highway, endangering the lives of the unsuspecting public.

Whenever we were planning a protest at a pain clinic, we would abide by the rules. We knew we couldn't block the entrance; we couldn't say anything to the clients. We would call beforehand to inquire if we needed a permit. Law enforcement knew we were going to be there. When the municipality was Broward County Police or Hollywood, we felt the officers were there to protect us. We never got that sense from Fort Lauderdale.

The 2014 Raid and Closure

Clinic owner charged with running $15 million pill mill - WSVN-TV - 7NEWS Miami Ft. Lauderdale: Carmel on the Case

Posted: Jun 05, 2014 6:15 PM EDT Updated: Jun 16, 2014 11:31 PM EDT Reported by Carmel Cafiero, Investigative Reporter

Produced by Daniel Cohen, Special Projects Producer

Joel Shumrak, owner of a South Florida pain clinic, is accused of writing prescriptions for trouble, supplying out of state dealers and drug addicts with some popular pain pills. Investigative reporter Carmel Cafiero has the exclusive.

FORT LAUDERDALE, Fla. (WSVN) – According to federal authorities, $15 million in pain pills traveled through the Pain Center of Broward and into the hands of addicts and drug dealers in Kentucky. 7Skyforce hovered over the scene on Tuesday, as the Fort Lauderdale clinic was raided, and the clinic's owner, Joel Shumrak, was arrested. The sixty-six-year old is accused of running a pill mill.

Carmel Cafiero, WSVN

"Thank you, God, that the DEA in Kentucky worked in conjunction with our DEA and closed them down," said Janet Colbert of STOPPNow, a group that rallies against pill mills.

Activists have protested at the clinic for years and consider Shumrak's arrest a success.

Maureen Kielian, also of STOPPNow, asked, "My question is that now that this clinic's closed, what about the doctors? Because you can't have a pill mill without a physician. They are the root of the problem. Florida has failed its citizens."

The mother who carried her daughter's ashes at the protests waited over three years for the arrest of Joel Shumrak and to see the eviction notice on the door of Pain Center of Broward. The clinic owner and a guard would stand out there and watch us at each protest. Shumrak thought it would never end. Although I spent many of my days off from work pacing up and down that sidewalk, I too thought he would never see the inside of a cell.

Joel Shumrak's Pain Clinic of Broward was only one of the pain clinics in Broward County, Florida. The sale of oxycodone was going well for the drug companies. The peddling of their product was paying off enormously. They also have been successful in blaming the deaths on the person who died – and the shortage of oxycodone on the DEA. There is a direct correlation between the increasing amount of oxycodone sales and the growing amount of deaths from oxycodone.

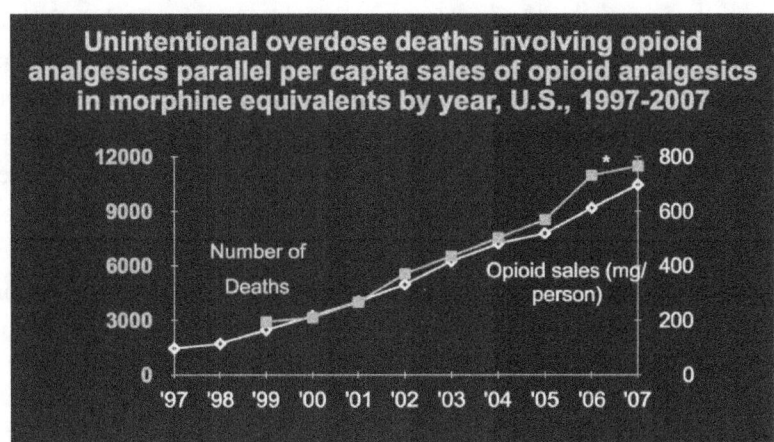

Note the increase of opioid deaths yearly. An increase in heroin deaths will later be seen due to the negligence of our legislators. Eight out of ten heroin addicts started with the opiate oxycodone. Source: National Vital Statistics System, multiple cause of death dataset, and DEAARCOS. *2007 opioid sales figure is preliminary.

The DEA crackdown below is in answer to correcting the malfeasant behavior contributing to the deaths. Regardless of the excessive number of pills being dispensed for no legitimate reason, it is the DEA who will later be blamed for the shortage of oxycodone.

U.S. Department of Justice

Drug Enforcement Administration

September 13, 2012

IN THE MATTER OF

Walgreen Co.
15998 Walgreens Drive
Jupiter, Florida 33478

ORDER TO SHOW CAUSE AND IMMEDIATE SUSPENSION OF REGISTRATION

Since at least 2009, the State of Florida has been the epicenter of a notorious, well-documented epidemic of prescription drug abuse. In July 2011, the Florida Surgeon General declared a Public Health Emergency based on the prescription pill epidemic, which results in an average of seven overdose deaths per day in Florida. The drugs most commonly associated with this epidemic are typically prescribed at unscrupulous pain clinics by physicians acting outside the usual course of professional practice and include Schedule II pain relievers, such as oxycodone; Schedule IV benzodiazepines, such as alprazolam; and Schedule IV muscle relaxers, such as carisoprodol (Soma). Frequently, these drugs are prescribed in large amounts and in combination with each other as "cocktails" popular with drug-seeking individuals.

Oxycodone is a dangerously addictive Schedule II controlled substance, which is known to be highly abused and diverted in the State of Florida. According to the 2010 Florida Medical Examiner's Commission Drug Report, the drug that caused the most deaths in the state of Florida for 2010 was Oxycodone (1,516 deaths).

According to DEA records, in 2011, Walgreens operated 7,862 retail pharmacies in the United States. Sixteen of the top twenty-five largest Walgreens retail in oxycodone purchasers, including the top six purchasers, were in Florida and supplied by Respondent. The following table shows these six stores and their yearly oxycodone purchases for 2009 through 2011:

Oxycodone Purchases by Dosage Unit

Florida

Store #	Location	2009	2010	2011
03629	Hudson	388,100	913,900	2,211,700
03099	Ft. Myers	95,800	496,100	2,165,900
06997	Oviedo	80,900	223,500	1,684,900
03836	Port Richey	344,000	849,000	1,406,000
04391	Ft. Pierce	250,000	881,400	1,329,600
04727	Ft. Pierce	153,500	507,100	1,192,000

Sales in all of the stores above increased dramatically in a two-year period. One store went from under 100,000 per year to over two million in one year. Oviedo, Florida, sold 1,684,900 in a town of only 34,00 residents, with only two Walgreens in the town. The police chief of Oviedo wrote letters to the pharmacies after each arrest made in their parking lots.

The Oviedo Police Chief convened a meeting with Walgreens Loss Prevention officials on February 10, 2011. He sent identical letters to both the Chairman and CEO of Walgreens asking them for their support and assistance in combating the prescription drug epidemic, informing them that Oviedo "has seen the parking lots of your stores become a bastion of illegal drug sales and drug use," where, once the prescriptions are filled, "the drugs are sold, distributed as payment, crushed and snorted, liquefied and injected, or multiple pills swallowed while in the parking lot of your pharmacies."

If we could control the greed of the high-prescribing doctors, there would still be plenty of pain pills (oxycodone) for patients who need them. Bear in mind though, oxycodone was never meant for chronic pain sufferers. There are more deaths now from oxycodone being taken *as prescribed* than there are from non-medical use. Many of those complaining that they must get their pills, and it is not fair that the drug addicts are ruining it for them, are, in fact, themselves addicted. It is the pill that is dangerous. It is highly addictive. The wrongdoer is not the person taking it, not the person becoming addicted to it.

Taken from the Annual Review of Public Health, December 29, 2014:

A Public Health Approach to an Epidemic of The Prescription Opioid and Heroin Crisis: Addiction

Andrew Kolodny, David T. Courtwright, Catherine S. Hwang, Peter Kreiner, John L. Eadie, Thomas W. Clark, and G. Caleb Alexander.

Over the past fifteen years, the rate of opioid pain reliever (OPR) use in the United States has soared. From 1999 to 2011, consumption of hydrocodone more than doubled and consumption of oxycodone increased by nearly 500 percent.

REFRAMING THE OPIOID CRISIS AS AN EPIDEMIC OF ADDICTION

Policy makers and the media often characterize the opioid crisis as a problem of nonmedical OPR abuse by adolescents and young adults. However, several lines of evidence suggest that addiction occurring in both medical and nonmedical users, rather than abuse per se, is the key driver of opioid related morbidity and mortality in medical and nonmedical OPR users.

Opioid Harms Are Not Limited to Nonmedical Users

Over the past decade, federal and state policy makers have attempted to reduce OPR abuse and OPR-related overdose deaths. Despite these efforts, morbidity and mortality associated with OPRs have continued to worsen in almost every U.S. state. Thus far, these efforts have focused primarily on preserving access to OPRs for chronic pain patients while reducing nonmedical OPR use, defined as the use of a medication without a prescription, in a way other than as prescribed, or for the experience or feeling it causes. However, policy makers who focus solely on reducing nonmedical use are failing to appreciate the high opioid-related morbidity and mortality in pain patients receiving OPR prescription for medical purposes.

The incidence of nonmedical OPR use increased sharply in the late 1990s, peaking in 2002 with 2.7 million new nonmedical users. Since 2002, the incidence of nonmedical use has gradually declined to 1.8 million in 2012. Although the number of new nonmedical users has declined, overdose deaths, addiction treatment admissions, and other adverse public health outcomes associated with OPR use have increased dramatically since 2002.

OPR overdose deaths occur most often in adults ages 45-54, and the age group that has experienced the greatest increase in overdose mortality over the past decade is 55-64, an age group in which medical use of OPRs is common. Opioid overdoses appear to occur more frequently in medical OPR users than in young nonmedical users. For example, in a study of 254 unintentional opioid overdose decedents in Utah, ninety-two percent of the decedents had been receiving legitimate OPR prescriptions from health care providers for chronic pain.

The proven evidence is there. We need measures that will result in fewer pills. No one should suffer, but the opiate is not the answer.

a Past month nonmedical OPR use by age

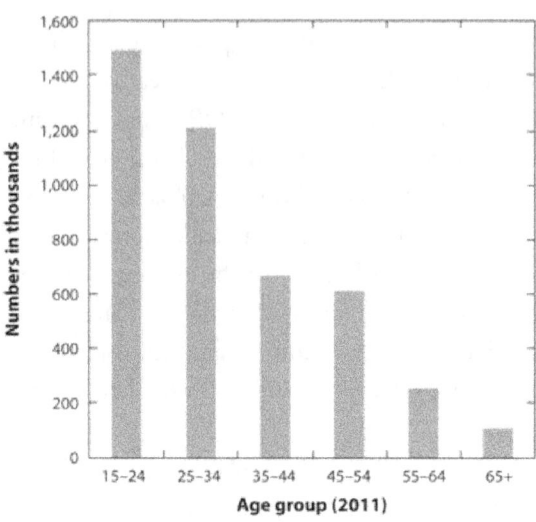

Kolodny A, et al. 2015.
Annu. Rev. Public Health. 36:559–74

b OPR-related unintentional overdose deaths by age

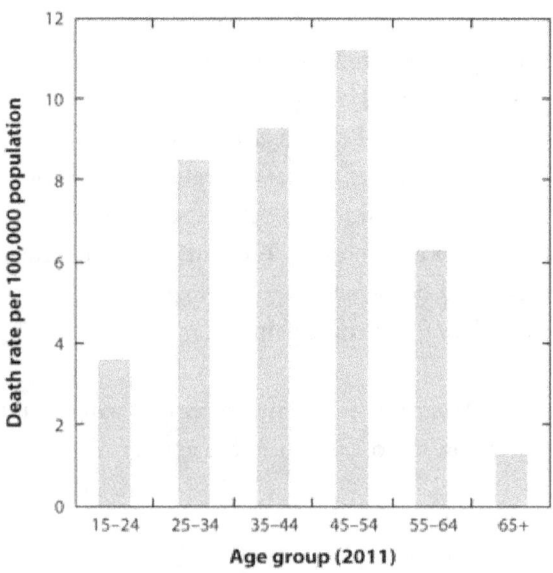

CHAPTER EIGHT

Legislation Needed: Is Anyone Listening?

Suckers for punishment that we are, and armed with our renewed exhilaration after the closing of Joel Shumrak's pill mill, on June 10, 2014, we sent an email to Senator Sobel requesting that we meet with her. This is the same Florida senator with whom we had had a conference call earlier and who expressed no interest in strengthening the PDMP (Not too much interest in humanoids either. But we were willing to try again.).

We explained that we need a legislative effort and/or bill to help save lives. We sent a link regarding the latest DEA raid in Broward County (the taking down of Joel Shumrak). We wrote about the fact that the pill mills still exist, and that the physicians are still prescribing. We were granted our meeting with Senator Sobel.

On June 25, 2014, at 4:00 p.m., we met Senator Sobel in her Hollywood, Florida, office. We spoke about all the continuance of deaths from the prescribed opiates. Senator Sobel asked, "what do you want me to do?" I said we would like her to write and sponsor a bill mandating the PDMP for prescribers of opiates and for Florida to be a part of the interstate exchange. Her response was, "I can do that." Senator Sobel said we could work with her legal assistant, Yale, to get the bill written.

Go figure. We were shocked and ecstatic. She had changed her mind. Perhaps it was the timing. The 2014 midterm elections were looming, and it was reported that the democrats were not expected to do well. We began canvassing the state for support. We sent Yale information regarding other states and the language used to write the bill.

> From: Janet Colbert stoppnow@yahoo.com
> Subject: PDMP
> Date: June 26, 2014
> To: Yale Olenick
>
> Yale:
>
> It was very nice meeting with you yesterday. Please thank Senator Sobel, as well. I am attaching Bill S 1657 [introduced 113th Congress by Senator Udall of New Mexico. A BILL to reduce prescription drug misuse and abuse] and a few items that may be of interest.
>
> Do you think we should leave the Narcan off of this bill due to its controversy, which there shouldn't be? I've administered it many times to newborn infants who are born not breathing. Different scenario – these are not the addicted babies, just got a little of the narcotic during the delivery process. It's a very good and safe drug, but I want to make sure the bill is going to be passed to strengthen the PDMP.
>
> Talk to you soon,
> Janet Colbert
> STOPPNow

Starting in August, we weren't hearing from Senator Sobel's office. We did ask repeatedly to speak with her office, both by leaving messages on voicemail and email. I did not hear back from their office.

> From: Stoppnow@yahoo.com
> Subject: PDMP
> Date: August 29, 2014
> To: Yale Olenick
>
> Yale:

We have been trying to contact you in regards to the bill to strengthen the PDMP. We have a few meetings scheduled next week to meet with legislators to garner support for its passage. Please contact us.

STOPPNow

At some point, you have to realize that when you give your word to someone, it does not hold the same meaning for all. Despite our efforts to gain endorsements throughout the state for the bill, we needed another plan. Maureen and I attended an open house hosted by Senator Maria Sachs on Thursday, January 15, 2015. Senator Sachs thanked her constituents for coming and explained a little about herself. Many were standing in line to speak to her. We were able to get a moment of her time to plead our case. Senator Sachs agreed to have a meeting with us to discuss a bill. Time for submitting a bill was running out. But she agreed to try to help.

Nine days later, on January 24, 2015, I wrote the following blog post on STOPPNow.com and sent it out to my STOPPNow contacts, which included Yale Olenick, Senator Sobel's assistant:

We had a "Hail Mary" pass yesterday.

We received a call from Senator Maria Sachs's office late yesterday afternoon. Senator Sachs put a bill into drafting to mandate the PDMP usage for prescribers of narcotics. Unlike Senator Eleanor Sobel, she kept her promise to us and did not give in to pressure from the powerful medical associations in Florida. Our task was that we had one hour to meet the deadline for filing a draft, and we needed someone from the House side to file the draft. Representative Evan Jenne's office filed that for us. We beat the deadline by ten minutes. We need more legislators who will put the needs of the people before their need to hold public office. Of course, without that distinction, they should not be holding public office.

This is only a draft. So now our work is cut out for us. We will work to get the bill written and passed. We ask that all of you call your Florida senators and representatives to express your support for this initiative. DRAFT #49588

All of a sudden we heard from Senator Sobel's office.

> From: Yale Olenick
> To: Stoppnow@yahoo.com
> Date: January 24, 2015
>
> FYI, the only reason your "Hail Mary" worked was the language that we helped craft and the coordination with our office and Sachs's at the last minute. Don't be hurt because we have other priorities like elderly abuse and neglect, children deaths, abuse and neglect … the list continues. I told your organization that it has nothing to do with industry pressure and is prioritizing our efforts and not being spread too thin. This blog post isn't fair, and is in fact just slander. It's best not to make enemies when you need as many friends as you can get.
>
> Yale Olenick

> From: Stoppnow@yahoo.com
> To: Yale Olenick
> Date: January 24, 2015
> Re: STOPPNow Blog
>
> Our phone calls stopped being answered, our emails unanswered. I think a human life is more important than greyhounds. I do appreciate your help though, and hope you can accept that. There was no slander there, only the truth.
>
> Janet Colbert
> STOPPNow

> From: Yale Olenick
> To: Stoppnow@yahoo.com
> Re: STOPPNow Blog

We're dealing with much more then greyhound lives in our office, Janet. You made a statement that was untrue in a public light. That's slander. Look it up. You have no evidence whatsoever to substantiate what you said. You were borderline harassing our office after I told you that we weren't going to sponsor it. I like to deal with professionals, not overzealous amateurs. I hope you can accept that too.

This last email from Yale Olenick was unsigned. I did not answer it, nor did I speak to Senator Sobel's office again. It seemed nonsensical to continue. We had sent nine emails in the eight-month time span in which communication stopped from their office. I never received any notice, written or by phone, that they decided to change their mind and not sponsor or try to gain support for the bill. That simple message would have ended it.

We have learned a lot along the way – much of it the hard way. All bills must go into drafting first, and there is a deadline. Senators can sponsor an unlimited number of bills, but, understandably, each bill presents a lot of work in order for it to move through to passage. The Florida House of Representatives are only permitted to sponsor six bills per session. We were not able to get a legislator from the House to sponsor the bill. They had either already sponsored their quota, or they weren't interested. We naively thought we had finally gotten the support we needed. So, another year goes by without needed legislation. And the deaths continue.

CHAPTER NINE

Still Work to Be Done

By the end of January, 2015, we realized that no Florida law strengthening the PDMP was going to take place this year. There was still work to be done.

We attended the Rockers in Recovery event held in Broward County on Valentine's Day, February 14, 2015. Rockers in Recovery hosts events throughout the United States to bring awareness to the prescription-drug epidemic. A host of speakers attend as well. Their website states that all who are seeking great music, sober fun, and addiction-recovery education are invited.

The talent in this group is beyond words. We also had a beautiful South Florida day. The sun was shining through the bluest sky, while the band played in the background, and people danced, lay on blankets, and threw Frisbees. It was a perfect day.

STOPPNow had a table set up to gather signatures for support of Naloxone. Naloxone is a drug antagonist against a narcotic. It is safe for use to bring back someone that has just overdosed. The bill would allow first responders, as well as third parties, to carry and administer Naloxone in the event of an overdose.

STOPPNow is also a member of a committee on substance abuse through the United Way of Broward County. Their white sheet concerning the latest data in Florida reads as follows:

In 2013, the most current reporting year, 4,781 people died in Florida with heroin or prescription drugs used non-medically in their systems. Altogether, there were 1,147 occurrences of heroin or morphine and 4,137 other opiates (narcotic pain relievers) detected in the 4,781 decedents.

All of these deaths were preventable. Often, when an individual overdoses, those who are with them may be afraid to contact the police or call 911 for fear they will be arrested for drug possession. However, Florida operates under the Good Samaritan Act, wherein any individual who acts in an emergency to provide help to someone in need of medical assistance will be granted immunity from any civil or criminal charges, including opiates. Family and friends should be aware of the Good Samaritan Act and contact 911 in the event of an overdose without fear of being arrested themselves.

Currently 29 states have enacted laws to provide for access and administration of Naloxone. Many states also have enacted Good Samaritan laws. Check in your state.

As people were stopping by our booth, I was telling them about the petition for Naloxone in our state. They were eager to sign. Many explained to me that Naloxone had saved their life. Some counted the number of days they have been in recovery, some in years. I hope and pray they all can win that struggle. These same individuals expressed agreement that doctors have shared responsibility in this epidemic. We are also still trying to have legislation passed to mandate that the prescriber check the database before writing a prescription for an opiate. In other states, these two measures have proven effective in saving lives.

Some stopped by and told me of the deaths of their children, husbands, and friends. These aren't just numbers. The suffering of those left to try to grasp why this happened to their loved ones was evident as they spoke. One woman told me that, as her daughter lay in a coma, she had a dream about her daughter being whole and beautiful. Her daughter did not survive. After the death of her daughter, this mother felt the dream was not to let her know her daughter would be OK in this life, but that she is now happy and at peace in the next.

When I left the concert, I went to mass. The gospel was about the lepers and how they were treated by society. They were to yell, "Unclean, unclean," if anyone approached them. One leper did approach Jesus and asked to be healed. Jesus reached down and touched him and he was healed. I sat in mass, having just left the concert, and thought how prophetic this sermon was on this day.

Many in our society blame the addict and do not want them to be a part of our society. But so many were not addicts until the drug companies got hold of them. The deceptive marketing tactics of the drug companies continue today. The drug companies have the added bonus that it is accepted belief that the addicts' deaths occurred because they were nothing but drug addicts. We need to change that. We need to place responsibility where it belongs. The drug companies and some doctors place more value on the almighty dollar than on human life.

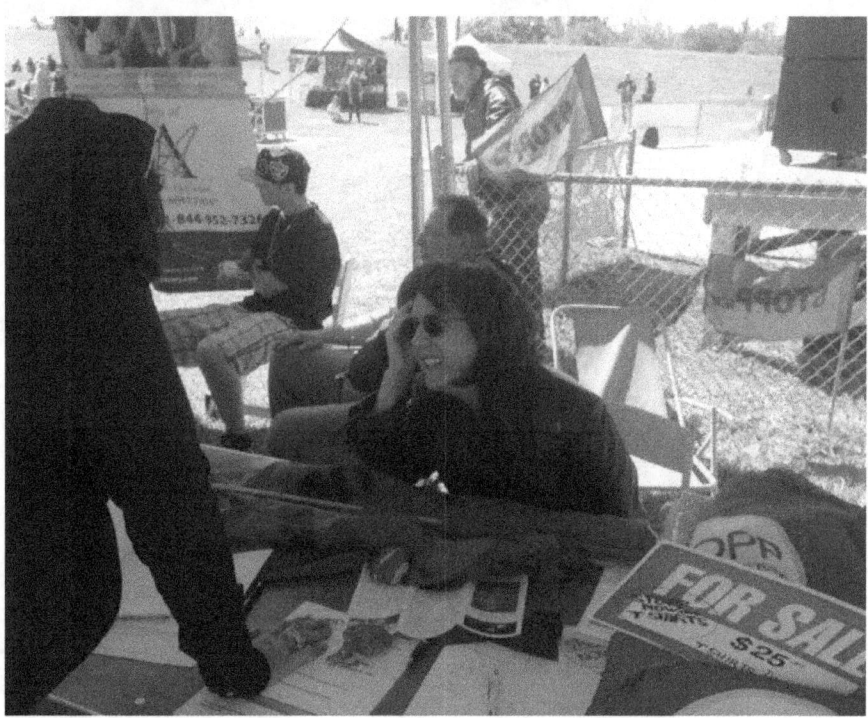

Janet of STOPPNow at Rockers in Recovery Event

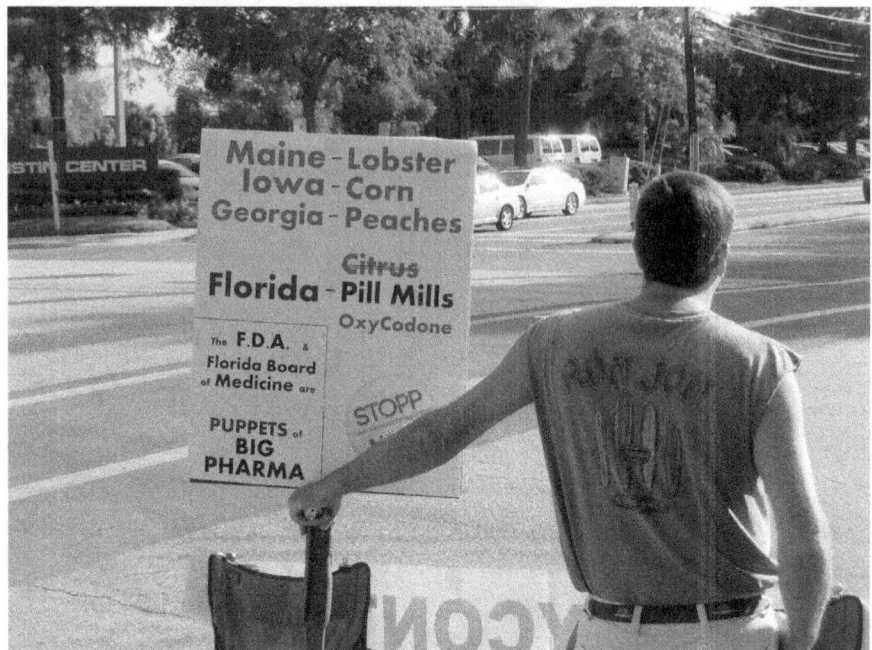

BOM Peaceful Protest

The next day, I wrote this letter to the Inspector General's office in the state of Florida:

February 15, 2015

Mr. Rob Beitler
Office of Inspector General
4052 Bald Cypress Way
BIN A03
Tallahassee, Florida 32399

Dear Mr. Beitler:

Thank you for taking the time to discuss the important matter of prescription drug deaths in our state and what can be done to change this. Too many parents are burying their children.

In 2013, the most current reporting year, **4,781 people died in Florida** with heroin or prescription drugs used non-medically in their systems. All together there were 1,147 occurrences of heroin or morphine and 4,137 other opiates (narcotic pain relievers) detected in the 4,781 decedents.

The Board of Medicine (BOM) could have and should have prevented this epidemic from occurring. Instead the deaths are mounting and the greed is allowed to flourish. A pill mill could not operate without a doctor with a license.

STOPPNow would like to propose that the BOM be audited every six months regarding complaints against a high opiate prescriber. The audit could be conducted by the drug court judges as they are faced every day with the result of non-restricted prescribing. We realize that the addict has some responsibility in this situation but the doctor plays a major role in what has been allowed to continue in our state.

STOPPNow was created due to the drug-addicted babies I was caring for as a Neonatal Intensive Care Nurse at Joe DiMaggio Children's Hospital. At the same time, my friend's son, under the influence of opiates, walked in front of a car on State Road 7 and was killed. The day before he had visited Vincent Coangello's pain clinic. At the time of his arrest, Vincent Coangello was making $150,000 a day. To date none of the doctors in that clinic have been arrested or lost their license to practice in our state.

I look forward to hearing from you. I would like to arrange a meeting with yourself and the Inspector General to discuss solutions to this ongoing tragedy in our state.

Sincerely yours,
Janet Colbert,
STOPPNow

Their response:

Florida HEALTH
Rick Scott
Governor

Mission: To protect, promote & improve the health of all people in Florida through integrated State, county, & community efforts.

Vision: to be the Healthiest State in the Nation

John H. Armstrong
State Surgeon General & Secretary

February 11, 2015

Janet Colbert

Dear Ms. Colbert

The Office of Inspector General (OIG), Florida Department of Health (DOH) carefully reviewed your concerns. The DOH remains interested in reducing substance abuse within the state of Florida. One tool that has been implemented is the Florida Prescription Drug Monitoring Program (PDMP), known as E-FORCSE (Electronic-Florida Online Reporting of Controlled Substance Evaluation Program). This program is intended to encourage safer prescribing of controlled substances and reduce drug abuse and diversion within the state of Florida. Florida statutes require that health care practitioners report to the PDMP each time a controlled substance is dispensed. [That would be the pharmacist who fills the prescription; the physician does not have to utilize this well-placed system].

The OIG has jurisdiction to investigate alleged violations of statute or policy pertaining to DOH entities. The OIG does not have statutory authority to review the medical or legal merits of practitioner complaints or act as an appeals tribunal for disputed Florida Board of Medicine Decisions.

By copy of this letter, we are forwarding your concerns to Lucy Gee, Director, Division of Medical Quality Assurance and Andre Ourso, Executive Director, Florida Board of Medicine.

No further action will be taken by this office.

Sincerely
James D. Boyd /CPA, MBA
Inspector General

cc: Lucy Gee, Director of Medical Quality Assurance
Andre Ourso, Executive Director, Florida Board of Medicine

The deaths continue, and it doesn't seem anyone has the job of changing that, but rather simply to state that the problem is resolved. The 2015 Medical Examiners Report can be found in the epilogue. From it, you will see that the problem is far from resolved.

We held a peaceful protest at the BOM meeting in September 2011. While traveling to Tampa, Florida, where it was held, I received an email from a person who asked that I call him regarding all of the work we have been doing. I called and he identified himself as Craig Turturo. He told me he was a fireman and wanted to help us.

His motivation, he said, was that he knew a person who had lost their life as the result of a pain clinic. He inquired how we came about knowing which pain clinics to protest in front of. Being the trusting soul that I am, I told him we have our ways. He said he had a lot of information regarding the BOM and how, even after suspending a license, they are reissued in another part of the state. He was willing to uncover all, but wanted to remain anonymous, as he was afraid.

I told him he could send me what he had, and I would pass it on. He was also willing to give me information on which pain clinics we should protest. He sent me some information. But then I saw a very small piece in the newspaper about two firemen who were charged with a misdemeanor for placing signs along a roadway in Naples, Florida. The signs were advertising their pain clinic in Miami. One of them was named Craig Turturo. I sent that to Craig and asked if he had seen it and told him that I had. I did not have any further correspondence from him.

It seems my new informant friend had been arrested and charged with drug trafficking and racketeering.

Two Pompano Beach firefighters arrested in pain clinic crackdown

June 27, 2012, Juan Ortega, *Sun Sentinel*

Operation Pill Street Blues: a multi-agency crackdown on a statewide network of illegal pain clinics.

Federal authorities alleged that firefighters Lewis Gabriel Stouffer, 32, of Coconut Creek, and Craig Louis Turturo, 32, of Boca Raton, were among a group of partners who made millions of dollars from pill mills.

Stouffer maintained a rapport with local law enforcement. He educated his co-conspirators on how to successfully report their competition as well as how to report doctor shoppers in order to appear as though they were legitimate pain clinics.

In recent months, one pill-mill suspect allegedly called Stouffer to alert him of the death of Forrest Cyphers, a patient of Dr. Roger Lee Gordon at Stuart Pain Management. Stouffer told him not to worry, as "people die every day."

CHAPTER TEN

We Just Don't Know When to Give Up

The number of babies born into addiction continued to rise. I decided to contact Andrew Benard, Assistant Deputy Attorney General and Special Counsel for the Florida Attorney General. I had met Andrew Benard on my earlier trip to Tallahassee.

> From: Janet Colbert
> Subject: CC Investigates Rise in Opioid-Addicted Newborns
> Date: March 10, 2015
> To: Andrew Bernard
>
> They're not recommending states to follow Florida's procedures on this.
>
> Janet Colbert
> STOPPNow

I included the CDC Report in the email. I will condense the report here:

> Nearly all of the infants with confirmed cases of neonatal abstinence syndrome (NAS) identified in three Florida hospitals during a two-year period had documented in utero opioid exposure. Yet only ten percent of their mothers received or were referred for drug addiction rehabilitation or counseling at the time of their infants' birth.

The researchers sought to identify maternal and infant characteristics in confirmed cases of NAS in Florida, where the number of hospital discharges of NAS-diagnosed infants has increased more than tenfold since 1995, far exceeding the threefold increase observed nationally.

The investigators identified three hospitals in two Florida counties with a high number of NAS births. From 2010 to 2011, a total of 242 infants with confirmed NAS were born in these hospitals. Of these, 99.6 percent of the infants were exposed to opioids in utero and 97.1 percent were admitted to an intensive care unit. Their mean length of stay was 26.1 days.

I sent a second email to schedule a phone call.

From: Janet Colbert
To: Andrew Bernard
Date: March 1, 2015
Subject Re: CDC Investigates Rise in Opioid-Addicted Newborns

Andrew:

They have recommended in the past to follow Florida's lead. This does not reflect well on Florida and is what I have been trying to do something about since I first starting writing. And you were the one answering my letters. These infants are still in trouble. The report did not say if these babies are going home with these mothers, without any help overcoming the addiction. This is, of course, a real danger to the infant found later, often too late. Would you be available on Thursday for a call?

Thank you,
Janet Colbert
STOPPNow

———

From: Andrew Benard
To: Janet Colbert
Date: March 10, 2015, at 12:56 PM

I'm available Thursday after 10:30 for the rest of the day.

Andrew Benard

I conferenced Maureen in on the phone call at the agreed time. At first, Andrew Bernard was very defensive. Understandably. They are getting blasted on all sides. And the report from us was that *You are not doing enough.* There are those who are contacting them because they feel the government is too involved and has no right telling them what to do. Others are calling complaining that they are suffering from chronic pain and cannot get the pills they need. We hear this from every legislative office we contact. There was a lot of venting. We spoke to him for an hour, and about midway through he said, "You know you are doing a lot, and you're not getting the respect you deserve."

He told us about how the Attorney General, Pam Bondi, had recently been getting her hair done in Tampa and noticed the shop next door. The goings on were indicative of a pill mill. The Attorney General took pictures and sent them to the proper authorities to investigate.

I told Andrew Bernard of the last pill mill where we protested, Prieto Medical Centers Mind and Body Wellness Center, 4242 N. Federal Highway, Fort Lauderdale. The pill mills have always been cash-only businesses. Very smart of them. Otherwise, the insurance companies would have shut them down a long time ago. But when we pulled up, we saw, in large letters across the plate glass window, *We accept all major insurance.*

Some were asking me, "Janet are you sure about this place?" But then, sure enough, the surrounding businesses came out, as they often do. "Thank God you're here." "They have fights in front of our establishments; we think they're coming through our windows." "We find hypodermic needles all over our sidewalks." When I inquired about the sign regarding acceptance of insurance they said, "He just put that up yesterday."

We went on to explain to Andrew Benard that the pill mills are still here; they are just not as blatant as they used to be. Gone are the days when there were ten pages advertising pill mills in the *New Times*. Dr. so and so has left; no more questions asked; etc. We explained that the pill mills are still here; they are just more cautious now.

I told Andrew Bernard that the BOM should be held accountable for their inaction. I told him also that they should be audited every six months regarding the outcome of any high-prescribing doctor that came before them for review. The audit could be conducted by the drug court judges because standing before them every day is the result of the BOM doing nothing to the real drug dealers. We told him how we are trying to get the PDMP mandatory for all prescribers to check prior to writing a prescription. This was stated during the venting phase of the conversation.

He told us, with great condemnation in his voice, that there are those who are trying to do away with the PDMP all together. Funding has been a problem for the PDMP since its inception, and now we think we can get something like this through?

Maureen said the mandate could be put on the BOM statutes. The prescribers would have to abide by it when applying for the DEA license and renewal.

All of a sudden, as I mentioned, Andrew Benard said, "Send me all of the things you have been telling me about. I will walk over personally to the Surgeon General's office and see if I can arrange a meeting, and I will attend with you."

We waited to hear from him. I believed his intentions were good, and I hoped we could accomplish what we have set out to do.

> From: STOPPNow@yahoo.com
> Subject: Prescription Drug Abuse
> Date: March 12, 2015
> To: Andrew Benard
>
> Andrew:
>
> Thank you so much for taking the time to speak to us. I included a letter I wrote to the Inspector General because it does state in writing that I would like an audit of the BOM. We are holding a Peaceful Protest at the

next BOM meeting. We would like to have a meeting with the Surgeon General to discuss holding the BOM accountable and making real change in this epidemic.

Thank you for all you do.
God Bless,
Janet Colbert
STOPPNow

We were never granted a meeting or phone call with the Florida Surgeon General. The suffering from the opiate epidemic continues.

CHAPTER ELEVEN

Carol

We first met Carol when she came to one of our STOPPNow rallies after reading about our cause on the front page of the local newspaper. Prior to that protest, Carol had not left her house after the death of her son, Buzzy, from prescription drugs, for two years.

Carol did not have a cell phone, didn't have a computer. We would notify all of our contacts of our next peaceful protest via email. We would always make the phone call to Carol to tell her of our next protest, and she never missed one. Her car wasn't up to par, and if the trek to the protest was too long, she would meet at one of our homes and ride with us. Carol didn't have riches in the worldly sense, but she enriched my life.

Carol told me that coming to the protests helped her, because at least she felt like she was doing something. We would spend hours walking up and down the sidewalks in front of pill mills, and there was a great camaraderie among the parents. No one can truly understand the loss of a child like a parent suffering that same loss. Carol told me at the St. Patrick's Day Parade on March 8, 2014, that she still cried herself to sleep every night. Buzzy had died March 11, 2008.

Carol had driven to my house on April 10, 2015, for the BOM meeting peaceful protest. On our way to the protest, Carol told me she had been diagnosed with lung cancer. She had known for about a year. She was still smoking, and when I asked, "Are you going to quit smoking?" she answered, "Why would I quit now, Jan?"

She told the doctor that she refused chemotherapy or the removal of her lung. She witnessed her sister take both measures, only to lose her life. She refused any further testing, stating that she does not need or want to know the date when she will die. Her only request is that she not live in pain. Ironically, opiates were originally approved for pain from cancer only. Of course, their highly addictive nature is not a consideration in someone suffering from end-of-life cancer.

I told Carol that when she goes she is going straight up. She said to me that she looks forward to seeing her son and hopes that he is there waiting for her.

Carol was not a negative person to be around, by any means. A diagnosis of lung cancer was not the worst news this mother had ever suffered. This goodhearted mother, who was so caring of others, was told by a medical examiner, while inquiring about the death of her son, that he was a drug addict. That pain, too, was still with her. As I continue to rant, it is the highly addictive nature of these pills that is to blame, not the person who becomes addicted to them.

Carol did not want any fuss to be made over her. She did not tell many of her illness. Her best friend, Brenda, who lived in Tampa, was not told until after Carol's death. She didn't want to cause disruption to anyone else's life.

When Carol's sister, Marie, called to tell me of her death, it was as though I was talking to Carol on the phone. They sounded exactly alike. Marie told me there was no service, but she would come back down from New Jersey in a few months. Carol wanted all her friends to meet down on Hollywood Beach to share a funny story about her. One November day, we did meet down on Hollywood Beach. We formed a circle and each shared a remembrance of Carol. There were a lot of tears and a lot of laughter. Brenda, her best friend, was totally devastated. We had met Brenda at the BOM protest held in Tampa.

A young girl told of Carol taking her under her wing. The girl spoke of the time Carol drove her to her high school play when she was sixteen. Carol met the then-sixteen-year-old girl's boyfriend, who is now her ex-husband, that night, many years ago. On the drive home from the play, Carol said to the girl, "What a hemorrhoid he is." I laugh whenever I think of that. I can hear Carol saying that.

They all said how a great joy was extinguished when Buzzy died. Yet, Carol's and my paths did not cross until after the death of her son. A light still shone.

Her sister Marie told me, while out on the beach, what she had experienced the night of Carol's death. Marie stated that they were not very religious. After being with Carol that night, she went back to the Marriott on Hollywood Beach. About 4:00 a.m., the hospice nurse called to tell her Carol had died.

Marie told me she went out on the balcony, despite the tremendous thunderstorm. She said there was a big crack of thunder, and she heard Carol say, as clear as day, "I could kill you for what you did to me." I prayed that Carol would get to see her son again, and I believe she is with him now.

CHAPTER TWELVE

Smoke and Mirrors?

It is the suffering endured by those parents mentioned in the preceding chapters and by those I have never met that makes me keep going. I will continue to fight for them until we put an end to this epidemic, which was conceived of and promoted by the drug companies.

In my pursuit of legislative support for our cause, I found that, as part of a federal investigation, on May 8, 2012, a letter had been sent from the U.S. Senate to the CEOs of the following drug companies:

- Endo Pharmaceuticals
- Purdue Pharma
- Johnson and Johnson

A similar letter was also sent to the heads of several organizations that have allegedly received payments from the drug companies:

- CEO, Federation of State Medical Boards
- Executive Director, American Pain Foundation
- Director, Center for Practical Bioethics
- President, American Academy of Pain Medicine
- Executive Director American Pain Society.

The letter to Purdue included this:

In 2007, top executives from Purdue Pharma, the original manufacturer of OxyContin, one of the most notorious and heavily abused painkillers, "pleaded guilty ... in federal court to criminal charges that they misled regulators, doctors, and patients about the drug's risk of addiction and its potential to be abused.

In 2003, a GAO report pointed to Purdue's partnership with the Joint Commission on Accreditation of Healthcare Organization (JCAHO) as possible means for Purdue to have "facilitated its access to hospitals to promote OxyContin." The report revealed that Purdue "funded over 20,000 pain-related educational programs through direct sponsorship or financial grants" in addition to funding the Joint Commission on Accreditation of Healthcare Organization's (JCAHO) pain management programs.

The Senators also ask for accounting of all payments from 1997 to present. Bear in mind they are asking if payments were made to the Boards of Medicine by drug companies.

Any nurse can tell you that when JCAHO (a government agency) is conducting a survey in their hospital, it is a major concern. If a hospital does not pass a JCAHO inspection, the facility's accreditation can be denied. Reimbursement for Medicare and Medicaid can be pulled. Pain was instituted as the "fifth vital sign." The hospital that fails a JCAHO inspection would have to close its doors; they could not operate without reimbursement. Brilliant of the drug companies to allegedly orchestrate this. Follow the money trail.

A letter from the senators (dare I call it an investigation?) was also sent to the Federation of State Medical Boards. As with the Purdue letter, the contents of this letter were tailored to the State Medical Boards with this addition:

As part of our effort to understand the relationship between opioid manufacturers and non-profit health care organizations, please provide the following information:

1) Provide a detailed account of all payments/transfers received from all organizations that develop, manufacture, produce, market, or promote

the use of opioid-based drugs from 1997 to the present. For each payment identified, provide:

   i. Date of payment.

   ii. Payment description (CME, royalty, honorarium, research support, etc.).

   iii. Amount of payment.

   iv. Year-end or year-to-date payment total and cumulative total payments for each organization or individual.

   v. For each year a payment was received, the percentage of funding from organizations identified above relative to total revenue.

2) Identify any grants or financial transfers used to fund the production of the book *Responsible Opioid Prescribing* by Dr. Scott M. Fishman. Provide the date, amount, and source of each grant.

3) How much revenue was generated by sales of *Responsible Opioid Prescribing*?

4) List each state that has distributed copies of *Responsible Opioid Prescribing* and the number of copies distributed.

5) Provide the names of any people or organizations, other than Federation of State Medical Boards employees or Dr. Scott M. Fishman, involved in writing or editing the content of *Responsible Opioid Prescribing*.

   i. for each person or organization identified, list any financial transfers between the identified person or organization and the Federation of State Medical Boards.

   ii. For each individual or organization identified, provide a description of the involvement.

The book referenced above, *Responsible Opioid Prescribing: A Physician's Guide*, by Scott M. Fishman, M.D., states:

> The Federation of State Medical Boards (FSMB) has commissioned this book and is distributing it to physicians to offer clear and concise guidelines in managing the risks of pain management with opioids.

The book also states:

> Over the past decade, two important public health trends have become entwined like the twin serpents in the caduceus: (1) increasing clinical attention across all medical specialties to the undertreatment of pain, and (2) shifting patterns of drug abuse from illicit to prescription drugs – most notably a dramatic rise in diversion and non-medical use of opioid pain medications within the United States.

First, the undertreatment of pain, and then, second, it is the fault of the one dying. Again, brilliant marketing.

The letter written specifically to the American Pain Foundation includes the following:

> A network of national organizations and researchers with financial connections to the makers of narcotic painkillers… helped create a body of dubious information: favoring opioids that can be found in prescribing guidelines, patient literature, position statements, books, and doctor education. Specifically, a patient guide funded by three drug companies and available on the American Pain Foundation website states that "there is no ceiling does (sic) for opioids as long as they are not combined with other drugs such as acetaminophen." However, a 2011 *Archives of Internal Medicine* paper found that the risk of death for high-dose patients was three times greater than in lower-dose patients.

The reference is Percocet, which consists of 5 mg oxycodone/325 mg acetaminophen. This, in large quantities, can destroy the liver. This is opposed to 30 mg oxycodone, which, in large quantities can kill you. But, according to the American Pain Foundation, there is no ceiling on the dose for opioids. The letter also asks:

What corporation provided the "$200,000 in seed money" received to found the American Pain Foundation in 1997?

A report in *Pro Publica*, by Charles Ornstein and Tracy Weber, on May 8, 2012, bears this headline: "American Pain Foundation Shuts Down as Senators Launch Investigation of Prescription Narcotics."

Dr. Andrew Kolodny, for whom I have a great respect, is quoted in the article as saying,

> These groups, these pain organizations… helped usher in an epidemic that's killed 100,000 people by promoting aggressive use of opioids. What makes this especially disturbing is that despite overwhelming evidence that their effort created a public health crisis, they're continuing to minimize the risk of addiction.

These letters, so widely disseminated and signed by Senator Chuck Grassley and Senate Investigation Committee Chairman, Senator Max Baucus, would lead one to believe that our U.S. Senate is aware of what is taking place and intends to do something about it. However, note the date on the letter: May 8, 2012. For all of their slight differences, each letter requested a response by June 8, 2012. It is now the end of 2016. There has been no FBI investigation. There have been no representatives from the drug companies or those allegedly paid by the drug companies testifying before the U.S. Senate. Is it all just smoke and mirrors?

The corruption is there to view. What are they doing about it? The deaths continue to rise.

United States Senate

COMMITTEE ON FINANCE

WASHINGTON, DC 20510-6200

May 8, 2012

David P. Holveck
President and Chief Executive Officer
Endo Pharmaceuticals Holdings Inc.
100 Endo Boulevard
Chadds Ford, PA 19317

Dear Mr. Holveck:

     As Chairman and a senior member of the Senate Finance Committee, we have a responsibility to the more than 100 million Americans who receive health care under Medicare, Medicaid, and CHIP. As part of that responsibility, this Committee has investigated the marketing practices of pharmaceutical and medical device companies as well as their relationships with physicians and non-profit medical organizations.

     It is clear that the United States is suffering from an epidemic of accidental deaths and addiction resulting from the increased sale and use of powerful narcotic painkillers such as Opana and Percocet. According to CDC data, "more than 40% (14,800)" of the "36,500 drug poisoning deaths in 2008" were related to opioid-based prescription painkillers.[1] Deaths from these drugs rose more rapidly, "from about 4,000 to 14,800" between 1999 and 2008, than any other class of drugs,[2] killing more people than heroin and cocaine combined.[3] More people in the United States now die from drugs than car accidents as a result of this new epidemic.[4] Additionally, the CDC reports that improper "use of prescription painkillers costs health insurers up to $72.5 billion annually in direct health care costs."[5]

     In Montana, prescription drug abuse is characterized by the state's Department of Justice as an "invisible epidemic" killing at least 300 people per year and contributing to increases in

---

[1] Center for Disease Control, "Drug Poisoning Deaths in the United States, 1980-2008, NCHS Data Brief, No. 81, December 2011 at http://www.cdc.gov/nchs/data/databriefs/db81.pdf.
[2] Id.
[3] CDC Press Release, "Prescription painkiller overdoses at epidemic levels," November 1, 2011 at http://www.cdc.gov/media/releases/2011/p1101_flu_pain_killer_overdose.html.
[4] LA Times, "Drug deaths now outnumber traffic fatalities in U.S., data show," September 17. 2011 at http://articles.latimes.com/2011/sep/17/local/la-me-drugs-epidemic-20110918.
[5] International Business Times, "Prescription Painkiller Overdoses Cost Insurers $72.5 Billion Yearly: CDC," November 3, 2011 at http://www.ibtimes.com/articles/242437/20111103/prescription-painkiller-overdoses-cost-insurers-72-5.htm.

addiction and crime.⁶ The University of Montana Bureau of Business and Economic Research estimated that prescription drug abuse is costing the state $20 million annually in additional law enforcement, social services, and lost productivity.⁷

In Iowa, "the use of opioid painkillers such as hydrocodone and oxycodone has increased dramatically in the last decade," according to the Governor's Office of Drug Control Policy. Annual overdose deaths from opioids "increased more than 1,233% from 3 deaths in 2000 to 40 deaths in 2009."⁸ Data from Iowa's prescription drug monitoring program demonstrates that in 2010, 89,500,000 doses of hydrocodone and oxycodone were prescribed totaling nearly 40% of all controlled substance prescriptions.⁹

Concurrent with the growing epidemic, the *New York Times* reports that, based on federal data, "over the last decade, the number of prescriptions for the strongest opioids has increased nearly fourfold, with only limited evidence of their long-term effectiveness or risks" while "[d]ata suggest that hundreds of thousands of patients nationwide may be on potentially dangerous doses."¹⁰

There is growing evidence pharmaceutical companies that manufacture and market opioids may be responsible, at least in part, for this epidemic by promoting misleading information about the drugs' safety and effectiveness. Recent investigative reporting from the *Milwaukee Journal Sentinel/MedPage Today* and *ProPublica* revealed extensive ties between companies that manufacture and market opioids and non-profit organizations such as the American Pain Foundation, the American Pain Society, the American Academy of Pain Medicine, the Federation of State Medical Boards, and the University of Wisconsin Pain and Policy Study Group.

According to the *Milwaukee Journal Sentinel/MedPage Today*, a "network of national organizations and researchers with financial connections to the makers of narcotic painkillers…helped create a body of dubious information" favoring opioids "that can be found in prescribing guidelines, patient literature, position statements, books and doctor education courses."¹¹ For example, the *Sentinel* reported that the Federation of State Medical Boards, with financial support from opioid manufacturers, distributed more than 160,000 copies of a model policy book that drew criticism from doctors because "it failed to point out the lack of science supporting the use of opioids for chronic, non cancer pain."¹²

In a *ProPublica* story published in the *Washington Post*, the watchdog organization examined the American Pain Foundation, a "health advocacy" organization that received "nearly

---

⁶ See the Montana Department of Justice website at http://doj.mt.gov/prescriptionabuse/.
⁷ Bureau of Business and Economic Research, "The Economic Cost of Prescription Drug Abuse in Montana", June 2011 at http://mbcc.mt.gov/PlanProj/Projects/PDMP/Prescription%20Drug%20Abuse%2020110629.pdf.
⁸ Iowa Governor's Office of Drug Control Policy, "Iowa Drug Control Strategy: 2012," November 1, 2011 at http://www.iowa.gov/odcp/drug_control_strategy/Strategy2012.Final.pdf
⁹ Id.
¹⁰ NY Times, "Tightening the Lid on Pain Prescriptions," April 8, 2012 at http://www.nytimes.com/2012/04/09/health/opioid-painkiller-prescriptions-pose-danger-without-oversight.html.
¹¹ Milwaukee Journal Sentinel/MedPage Today, "Follow the Money: Pain, Policy, and Profit," February 19, 2012 at http://www.medpagetoday.com/Neurology/PainManagement/31256.
¹² Id.

90 percent of its $5 million funding from the drug and medical device industry."[13] *ProPublica* wrote that its review of the American Pain Foundation's "guides for patients, journalists, and policymakers play down the risks associated with opioids and exaggerate their benefits. Some of the foundation's materials on the drugs include statements that are misleading or based on scant or disputed research."[14]

Although it is critical that patients continue to have access to opioids to treat serious pain, pharmaceutical companies and health care organizations must distribute accurate information about these drugs in order to prevent improper use and diversion to drug abusers.

As part of our effort to understand the relationship between opioid manufacturers and non-profit health care organizations, please provide the following information:

1) Provide a detailed account of all payments from 1997 to the present between Endo and the following organizations in table format:

   a. Organizations
      i. The American Pain Foundation
      ii. The American Academy of Pain Medicine
      iii. The American Pain Society
      iv. The American Geriatric Society
      v. The Wisconsin Pain and Policy Study Group
      vi. The Alliance of State Pain Initiatives
      vii. The Center for Practical Bioethics
      viii. Beth Israel Medical Center, Department of Pain Medicine and Palliative Care
      ix. The Joint Commission (and all related entities)
      x. The Federation of State Medical Boards
   b. Individuals
      i. Russell K. Portenoy, M.D. – Chairman, Department of Pain Medicine And Palliative Care at Beth Israel Medical Center
      ii. Scott M. Fishman, M.D. – Chief, Department of Pain Medicine, University of California, Davis
      iii. Perry G. Fine, M.D. - Professor of Anesthesiology, Pain Research Center, University of Utah School of Medicine
      iv. Lynn R. Webster, M.D., F.A.C.P.M., F.A.S.A.M. – Medical Director and Founder, Lifetree Clinical Research & Pain Clinic
      v. Rollin M. Gallagher, M.D., M.P.H. – Director of Pain Management, Philadelphia Veteran Affairs Medical Center
      vi. Bill McCarber, M.D. – Founder of the Chronic Pain Management Program for Kaiser Permanente in San Diego, CA

---

[13] ProPublica, "The Champion of Painkillers," December 23, 2011 at http://www.propublica.org/article/the-champion-of-painkillers.
[14] Id.

vii. Martin Grabois, M.D. – President, American Academy of Pain Medicine
viii. Myra Christopher – Kathleen M. Foley Chair for Pain and Palliative Care, Center for Practical Bioethics

c. For each organization or individual identified in 1(a) and 1(b), provide:
   i. Date of payment.
   ii. Payment description (CME, royalty, honorarium, research support, etc.).
   iii. Amount of payment.
   iv. Year-end or year-to-date payment total and cumulative total payments for each organization or individual.

2) All documents and communications from 2004 to the present pertaining to the book, "Responsible Opioid Prescribing: A Physician's Guide," distributed by the Federation of State Medical Boards.
   a. Provide the names, titles, and job descriptions of all employees who collaborated with the Federation of State Medical Boards, Dr. Scott Fishman, or third-party contractors on the development of this book.
   b. For each employee identified in 2(a), provide a summary of the work performed pertaining to the book.

3) All documents and communications from 2007 to the present pertaining to the development or changes to JCAHO's[15] pain management standards, including but not limited to communications with the American Pain Society and other organizations involved in developing JCAHO pain management standards.

4) All documents and communications from 2007 to the present pertaining to the development or changes to The American Pain Society's pain guidelines.

5) All documents and communications from 2004 to the present pertaining to the American Pain Foundation's Military/Veterans Pain Initiative.

6) All documents and communications from 2007 to the present pertaining to any policies, guidelines, press releases and/or position papers distributed by the American Pain Foundation.

7) All presentations, reports, and communications to Endo's management team or board of directors from 2007 to the present pertaining to the funding of and/or collaborations with of any of the organizations or individuals specified in request 1(a) or 1(b).

---

[15] All requests pertaining to JCAHO include related organizations such as the "Joint Commission Resources."

In cooperating with the Committee's review, no documents, records, data, or other information related to these matters, either directly or indirectly, shall be destroyed, modified, removed, or otherwise made inaccessible to the Committee.

We look forward to hearing from you by no later than June 8, 2012. All documents responsive to this request should be sent electronically, on a disc, in searchable PDF format to my staff. If you have any questions, please do not hesitate to contact Christopher Law with Senator Baucus at (202) 224-4515 or Erika Smith with Senator Grassley at (202) 224-5225.

Sincerely,

Charles E. Grassley
Senator

Max Baucus
Chairman

CHAPTER THIRTEEN

More Smoke, More Mirrors

The effect of the opiate is not just in Broward County, Florida. However, Broward County holds the distinction of being the epicenter of the prescription drug epidemic in the United States. Other countries have been looking to the U.S. for answers.

I received an email requesting an interview with RT International News Channel. It is a Russia-based agency that delivers news in many languages to people around the world. The interviewer was interested in telling the story of the opiate due to the massacre that took place June 2015 in Charleston, South Carolina. I heard, too, about the shooter being on suboxone. Suboxone is a medical assisted treatment (MAT) for opiates. It can be a helpful drug; it can also be used in conjunction with opiates. As much as this epidemic is permeating and destroying our society, the opiate was not the reason for such hatred and pure evil.

Part of the news coverage for this act was that the murderer sat in that church for almost an hour before he shot and killed nine innocent people. It was also reported that his victims had been so kind that he almost changed his mind and did not go through with it. It's too bad he did not listen to that voice. How different his and the lives of many others could have been.

I agreed to tell the RTI interviewer the opiate story from my perspective. I believe that, as I spoke, the passion for what I was saying was obvious, but I feel so tired of telling the same story over and over. This has been going on for so many years, and we can't get anyone to end this accepted malady in our country. Just before the interview, I wrote to the U.S. Surgeon General, who serves as the principal advisor to the Secretary of Health and Human Services on public health and scientific issues, requesting a meeting, as I was going to be in Washington, D.C. for the FED Up Rally. I asked that he take ownership of this and not remain silent.

Recently, I attended a meeting that included some parents whose children were still facing addiction and others who had buried their children from addiction. One parent who lost her son a few months ago was tearfully explaining the loss and isolation they are feeling. According to a United Way of Broward County Commission on Substance Abuse Annual Drug Trends Report of June 2015, the number of prescription opioid crime laboratory reports increased eighty-seven percent between 2013 and 2014. The best answer would be to stop the production. The drug does more harm than good, which should be the catalyst for removing a drug from the market. Despite this fact, the opiate remains on the market, while the suffering of some – along with the wealth of others – continues.

And in another victory for the wealth side, just after I attended the above-mentioned meeting, the FDA approved 5 mg/5 ml formulation of oxycodone HCL liquid. Once while protesting outside a notoriously bad pain clinic, the business next door told us that customers of the pain clinic were constantly coming in and asking if they could use their microwave to warm up a baby bottle. They used to melt the pill on a teaspoon of hot water in order to shoot up. Well, that will no longer be necessary. Not now that the FDA has approved liquid oxy. Good job, FDA!

Businesses that were neighbors of the pain clinics were always glad to see us. They would tell us of hypodermic needles all over their sidewalks. Despite the law that no longer allows dispensing from pain clinics, this still went on without repercussions. A common complaint from small businesses in strip malls trying to make a living was that customers were afraid to visit their establishment due to what was going on next door at the pill mill. More than once, it was the businesses within the strip mall who would contact us and ask that we hold a protest. Of course, the BOM meetings were different. They were held in hotels. And they were not glad to see us. However, even after police were called, it was established we were allowed to be there, too.

Don't forget: This is a physician-prescribed epidemic, which the BOM could have prevented and could still now stop.

An international senate caucus was held in 2014. (This gave us another reason for hope. Yet, as of this writing, two-and-a-half years have gone by since this caucus and without lessening the amount of opiate produced. The deaths continue to rise, and babies continue to be born addicted to the opiate. We need more than just talk and feigned concern.)

The senators listened to testimony by Michael Botticelli, then Acting Director of the Office of National Drug Control Policy (ONDCP); Dr. Nora Volkow, Director of the National Institute on Drug Abuse; Dr. H. Westley Clark, Director of the Center for Substance Abuse Treatment; Joseph Rannazzisi, Deputy Assistant Administrator of the DEA; and Dr. Andrew Kolodny, then CMO of Phoenix House, who is an advocate for change.

United States Senate Caucus on International Narcotics Control held May 14, 2014

Prepared Statement of Co-Chairman, Senator Chuck Grassley

Senator Grassley signed the letter sent by the Senate Investigation in May 2012.

The complete hearing can be found on www.drugcaucus.senate.gov

> I'm glad that our hearing today will address both the abuse of heroin and prescription opioids. The two issues are linked. Once some people get hooked on prescription painkillers, they often turn to heroin, which is much cheaper.
>
> The abuse of these types of drugs is a problem that I have been concerned about for some time. In 2010, I worked with Senator Klobuchar to pass the Secure and Responsible Drug Disposal Act. This law allows for com-

munities to establish prescription drug "take back" programs, so patients can safely dispose of old or unused medicines.

Why not a law to produce fewer pills instead of throwing them away?

> Last year, Senator Feinstein and I learned about the existence of a database of doctors maintained by Purdue Pharmaceuticals. Purdue markets OxyContin, one of the most abused prescription opioids. The database allegedly contained information about doctors who engaged in reckless prescribing practices.

> Our investigation revealed that many state medical boards, as well as the Centers for Medicare and Medicaid Services, didn't know about this database. We encouraged these organizations, as well as the DEA, to contact Purdue about it. As a result, information is now in the hands of authorities who can take action against an irresponsible doctor.

Senator Dianne Feinstein Opening Statement

> Four out of every five heroin abusers had abused prescription pain relievers in the past. So, pain relievers like oxycodone and hydrocodone affect the central nervous system in much the same way as heroin. So, the lesson here is that rather than thinking of two separate addictions (prescription pain medications and heroin), we should realize we are facing a much larger opioid addiction epidemic that includes both.

I agree. The public would be better informed if an ER doctor, while treating a sprained ankle, asked, "Do you want some heroin for the pain."

> So, the strategy to battle these drugs should have three parts: preventing drug use, treating addicts, and reducing the number of overdoses. But the first and most important strategy is to prevent opioid drug [sic] before it starts.

I hate to sound like a broken record, but fewer pills would be the best way to accomplish this. Let's lower the production numbers.

Drug take back programs can also help reduce opioid abuse because they get unused prescription pain medicines out of family medicine cabinets, where too many young adults first obtain these drugs.

I wholeheartedly agree with the three strategies: preventing drug use, treating addicts, reducing overdoses. Senator Feinstein supported the Comprehensive Addiction and Recovery Act (CARA). CARA passed the U.S. Senate on March 10, 2016, by a vote of ninety-four to one. However, the mandate for the PDMP was removed. CARA authorized $181 million dollars each year in new funding to fight the opioid epidemic. Unfortunately, this is needed – but it will always be needed because no effort is being made to produce fewer pills. This will never end. The drug companies are making money on both ends. First they addict them; then they treat the addiction with medication-assisted treatment (MAT). Narcan is also a much-needed antidote to reverse an overdose. It's all more money for the drug companies, the biggest lobbyists.

Senator Amy Klobuchar was also in attendance at the hearing. This was taken from her website:

> In the last four years, up to four million pounds of prescription drugs have been collected across the country during designated prescription drug take back days.

Prescription drug take back will help keep the pills off the street – the already bought-and-paid-for drugs. At least Senator Amy Klobuchar is instituting measures into law that will help. Senator Klobuchar, along with Senator Joe Manchin and Senator Angus King, introduced S. 3209 Prescription Drug Monitoring Act of 2016. The bill requires the use of the PDMP and the facilitation of information sharing among states. (You can reach Senator Joe Manchin by email, if you would like to contact him: endtheopioidcrisis@manchin.senate.gov.)

We'll have to monitor the bill. I wasn't successful in getting Florida to bring this law to fruition. This, if passed, would make the requirement on a national level.

A letter was sent to Purdue Pharma on behalf of the Senate Caucus on International Narcotics Control on November 8, 2013. (Yet there was no mention made of the May 8, 2012, letter. The senators seem to be good at writing letters.) This is the result of the international caucus held in 2013.

I wrote to Senator Feinstein and asked that she not use the Senate Caucus on International Narcotics for political purposes. Maureen and I met once a week with an agenda for STOPPNow. We spoke to Senator Feinstein's and Senator Grassley's offices on many occasions. When we arrived for a pre-arranged meeting in Senator Feinstein's Washington, D.C. office with the drug caucus staff on September 30, 2014, we were welcomed into their conference room, where we presented facts regarding the deaths and suffering in our communities from the opiate. We were told they were waiting for the Government Accountability Office (GAO) Report before making any recommendations to Senator Feinstein.

After our allotted time in the conference room, we were escorted for further discussion out into the hallway. We were escorted past the reception area, which had a vacant couch and chairs, and were made to stand in the hall for the remainder of our presentation.

While in Washington, we also met with Congressman Marsha Blackburn's office. At that meeting, we were escorted out of Representative Blackburn's office and led into a small, locked room, little bigger than a closet, for our meeting. Karen L. Summar, Legislative Assistant to Congressman Blackburn, told the receptionist: "I'm taking them down to the annex for this meeting." I posted details of the meeting on a STOPPNow blog on October 6, 2014:

STOPPNow Blog

STOPPNow attended the FED Up Rally this weekend, September 28, 2014, and marched to the White House. Much needs to be done, as evidenced by the 2,000 in attendance and those also suffering loss who were not able to attend. The reception was held Saturday, September 27, 2014. As they were showing pictures of lost loved ones on a large screen, I could hear sobbing and see uncontrollable shaking from the young man seated next to Maureen. Mark was there from Massachusetts with his sister. They had just lost their mother four weeks earlier from the opiate epidemic. Mark said that the pills are still coming from Florida.

United States Senate

SENATE CAUCUS ON
INTERNATIONAL NARCOTICS CONTROL
HART SENATE OFFICE BUILDING, ROOM 818-C
WASHINGTON, DC 20510

November 8, 2013

Mr. John H. Stewart
President and Chief Executive Officer
Purdue Pharma L.P.
One Stamford Forum
201 Tresser Boulevard
Stamford, CT 06901-3431

Dear Mr. Stewart:

According to an August 11, 2013 *Los Angeles Times* article entitled "OxyContin Maker Closely Guards Its List of Suspect Doctors," Purdue maintains a list of doctors who are suspected of "recklessly prescribing" OxyContin to "addicts and drug dealers." The list, according to the article, was created as a way for Purdue to "steer its sales representatives away from risky doctors." Unfortunately, we understand that this list has not been made available to law enforcement, the Centers for Medicare and Medicaid (CMS), or state medical boards.

According to the Office of National Drug Control Policy, prescription drug abuse is our nation's fastest growing drug problem. The U.S. Substance Abuse and Mental Health Services Administration's *2012 National Survey on Drug Use and Health* (NSDUH) found that nearly 12.5 million individuals 12 years or older used pain relievers for non-medical reasons in 2012. The NSDUH report further indicates that past month abuse of prescription medications including pain relievers, tranquilizers, stimulants, and sedatives is second only to marijuana, the number one abused drug in the United States. Earlier this year, the Centers for Disease Control (CDC) reported that that drug overdose deaths increased for the eleventh straight year, with sixty percent of overdose deaths (22,134) involving pharmaceutical drug products and three-quarters of those deaths (16,651) involving oxycodone, hydrocodone, methadone and other opioid analgesics. For this reason, CDC has classified prescription drug abuse as an epidemic.

In a series of interviews conducted by the *Los Angeles Times*, a Purdue senior executive reported that your company trained its sales representatives to internally report "red flags" identifying suspect doctors. For example, a doctor would be flagged if the sales representative noticed "young patients, long lines, people nodding off in waiting rooms and frequent cash transactions." If Purdue determined that a doctor's practices appeared to be "too risky," Purdue would bar sale representatives from marketing to the doctor, stop paying commissions on his or her OxyContin prescriptions, and assign the doctor to the company's database referred to in the article as "Region Zero."

With regard to these doctors, as your senior executive indicated in the article, Purdue does not have "the ability to take the prescription pad out of their hand." However, Purdue does have the ability – if not the responsibility – to share this information appropriately with those who can do so. According to the article, Purdue has reported a mere 154 prescribers – or 8% of the 1,800 doctors in the database – to law enforcement or medical regulators. Therefore, it appears that Purdue has potentially valuable tips that it has not passed on to authorities relating to many other reckless doctors who may be fueling this epidemic of prescription drug abuse.

To help better understand Purdue's Region Zero database, please provide the following information by November 27, 2013:

1. The list of all doctors contained in the database, each of their Medicare provider numbers, and the information that triggered their assignment to the database.

2. The criteria Purdue uses to decide whether to report a doctor to law enforcement or medical regulators.

3. Any information known to Purdue regarding the results of any of its 154 referrals of doctors to law enforcement or medical regulators, including any arrests, indictments, convictions, license revocations, or any other enforcement actions.

4. Whether Purdue has provided the database or its contents to CMS or any law enforcement agency, and whether any law enforcement agency has subpoenaed it.

5. Whether Purdue has provided the database or its contents to any wholesalers with which it has a business relationship.

In addition, we call on Purdue to provide the Region Zero database to the Senate Caucus on International Narcotics Control, Drug Enforcement Administration, CMS, and appropriate state medical boards so the information contained in it may be reviewed for appropriate action.

Thank you very much for your attention to this matter. We look forward to your prompt response.

Sincerely,

Senator Dianne Feinstein
Chairman

Senator Charles Grassley
Co-Chairman

Senator Edward Markey

Senator Charles Schumer

Senator Tom Udall

We had scheduled meetings with offices of senators and representatives. One must wonder where the U.S. Surgeon General is in all of this. The CDC has named the prescription drug deaths to be a national epidemic for years, now. Gone are the days when we had a surgeon general speak out against irresponsible companies, like with Big Tobacco. Rear Admiral Boris D. Lushniak, M.D., M.P.H., is acting Surgeon General since 2013; no permanent appointment has been made. But he is not acting like a surgeon general. He is silent.

I must share one meeting that we had with Karen L. Summar, M.D., M.S., Legislative Assistant to Congressman Blackburn, 7th District Tennessee, U.S. House of Representatives. I asked Karen Summar if she could explain HR 4709, co-sponsored by Representative Blackburn and sponsored by Representative Tom Marino, 10th Congressional District Pa. (HR 4709 passed unanimously in the House.) We feel it ties the hands of the DEA.

She stated that, if a pharmacy makes one mistake, then the DEA is taking away their license. I asked if she could give us one example, since this is not the case in Florida. I had files with me pertaining to Walgreens and their Jupiter Distribution Center. They were cited for clear diversion of prescription drugs. Walgreen stores went from under 100,000 oxycodone purchases a year to over two million.

In addition, I stated that I had put one in particular aside for Representative Blackburn, as it directly relates to her bill. The Walgreens customer was issued too many pills by mistake. The store called the individual's house in an attempt to retrieve the pills. The store was told by the customer's girlfriend that he is a drug dealer and is out selling the pills and that he told his girlfriend that he hit pay dirt today. Despite this incident, the pharmacy continued to fill his prescriptions.

Ms. Summar took that Walgreens report. Maureen asked her how she felt about the PDMP. I said that we would like it to be mandatory. She abruptly stood, said, "This meeting is over," and left. Maureen and I looked at each other and asked what just happened. The meeting lasted less than five minutes and was hostile in nature. It was very bizarre; we gathered our things and walked out into the hallway. Our host, Representative Blackburn's assistant, was nowhere in sight.

The bill is now in the Senate as S-2862, sponsored by Senator Whitehouse and Senator Hatch. Changes have been made, and it is an improvement over HR 4709. However, it is still compromising to the DEA.

We met with the DEA in Arlington, Virginia, on Wednesday October 1, 2014. What a welcome change, totally different tone. I explained all of the above. Maureen is in Pennsylvania for a few more days and has been unable to obtain a meeting with Representative Marino's office.

We will be having a follow-up conference call with DEA. My goal is still to reduce production. We do not need 114 tons of pills.

I ask all of you to contact your state surgeon general's office and request to have the fifth vital sign, that of pain, to be removed; there does not need to be a standing order for a thirty-day supply of opiates for a post-op patient, nor for a large number of opiates being prescribed by dentists after extraction of wisdom teeth. The public perception of those not touched by this epidemic is to trust their doctor and take as prescribed. They are not aware that this is a highly addictive drug.

Stay tuned.

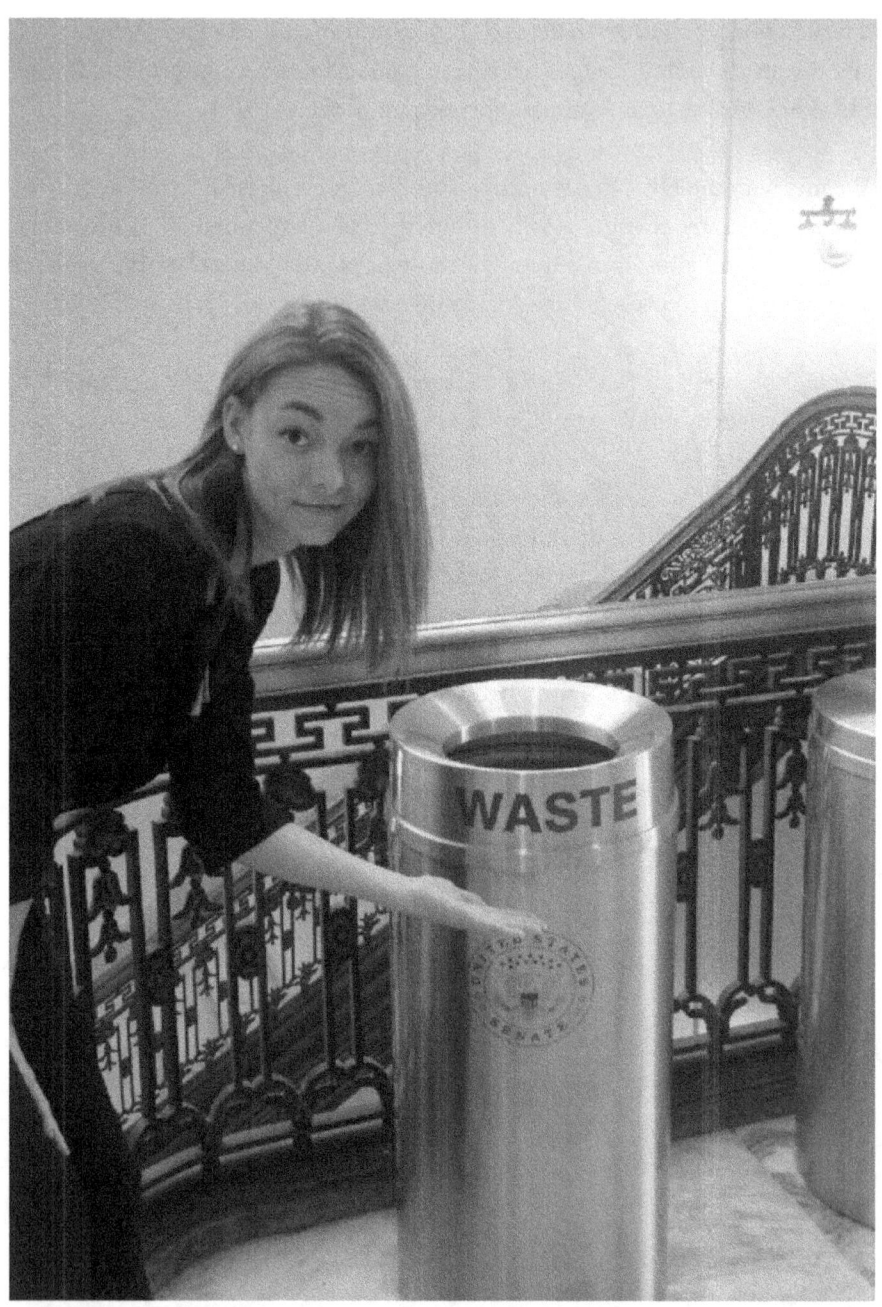

As we were walking down the steps of the Rayburn House Office Building still stunned by our meeting with Representative Blackburn's assistant I received this text from Shelby. Our fellow advocates were not faring any better over at the Senate offices (WASTE)

CHAPTER FOURTEEN

Yet Another Meeting

You have just read through the so-called "Senate Investigation" and the United States Senate Caucus on International Narcotics Control Hearing. Matters would seem to be in good hands. Or is it just talk? The GAO report, that Senator Feinstein's office told us they could not make any recommendations to the senator until its release, has been concluded.

Published in *DEA Chronicles*

Senate Committee Questions DEA on Quota Process

By Larry Cote on May 6, 2015

On May 5, 2015, the United States Senate Caucus on International Narcotics Control held a hearing exploring the findings and recommendations of a Government Accountability Office Investigation into the Drug Enforcement Administration's management of its quota process. The hearing, called by Senators Grassley and Feinstein, sought to explore the connection between DEA's quota process and pharmaceutical drug shortages in the United States.

At the hearing, DEA and the Food and Drug Administration announced that the agencies recently entered into a Memorandum of Understanding to facilitate collaboration between the agencies, including greater information sharing. While the hearing was generally cordial, Senator Whitehouse did press DEA on its historic failures to issue quota in a timely manner. Senator Whitehouse questioned whether DEA was able to effectively manage its administrative and regulatory responsibilities and whether those functions should be transferred out of DEA. Specifically, Senator Whitehouse noted that "dissatisfaction with DEA's level of capability and performance as an administrative regulator runs very deep and is very broad," and that DEA is running the risk of losing bi-partisan support on Capitol Hill.

This is their conclusion? The long-awaited GAO report? They decided it was more important to hold a senate hearing to investigate the DEA? Is it just me, or does this seem a little threatening? The DEA is being blamed for the shortage of pills. Yet, the senators who can put laws in place to stop the deaths from the opiate epidemic do not do so.

Senator Whitehouse blames the DEA for shortages of pain pills, and the deaths continue to rise. Interestingly enough, Senator Whitehouse represents the State of Rhode Island. CVS Pharmacy's corporate headquarters are located in Rhode Island. Maybe the DEA went too far and had to be brought to task for their infraction.

Read the story below, regarding a couple of CVS pharmacies in a little town known as Sanford, Florida.

WESH ORLANDO by Matt Grant

Sanford, Florida – Federal agents and CVS pharmacy officials are speaking out about a $22 million fine the chain received for its poor prescription drug practices in Florida. Under the agreement with the Department of Justice, CVS admits pharmacists knowingly filled thousands of illegitimate prescriptions for painkillers, mostly oxycodone, in Florida between 2010 and 2011. Katherine Ho, who is the assistant U.S. attorney for the Middle District of Florida, said CVS violated the Controlled Substance Act by failing to verify that the prescriptions, which came from pill mills, were legitimate. According to the DEA, the two locations were ordering one million to two million oxycodone pills a year, which is twenty-seven times the national average. Those locations' DEA licenses have been revoked, so they can no longer dispense narcotic medications.

Could there be any connection between this ridiculous amount of prescribing and the shortage? The accusations against the DEA for the shortage of pills is criminal in itself. If their time is spent defending their agency, they can't do their job effectively.

Let me tell you about the pharmacy crawl, also the DEA's fault: Florida was experiencing a "pharmacy crawl," which started at the same time the DEA was cracking down on pill mills and pharmacies dispensing oxycodone by the millions. Some legitimate pharmacists became fearful of losing their license. The news was full of pain patients who were not able to fill their prescriptions. This prompted them to go from pharmacy to pharmacy to try to get their pain pills, which became known as the "pharmacy crawl."

Pharmacists were in a tough spot. Doctors do not like being questioned by a pharmacist. On August 10, 2015, the Florida Board of Pharmacy Controlled Substances Standards Committee called a meeting. The public was invited, and each individual was allowed three minutes to speak. STOPPNow was in the front row with our red shirts to support the DEA.

When it was my turn to speak, I started by mentioning the fact that I was very disappointed that Nabil El Sanadi, M.D., Florida Board of Medicine, had left the meeting early and was not there to hear my presentation. Then I gave my presentation, including the material I had submitted to the committee before speaking:

> The DEA is here today to explain their action. I would like to thank the DEA and law enforcement for their part in trying to alleviate the crisis caused by the physician-prescribed epidemic in our country. The court documents are a matter of public record and describe why it was necessary for the DEA to raid the pharmacies in question.
>
> The court documents relating to the six pharmacies that are written earlier in this text were presented. The DEA approves the amount of oxycodone produced every year. We have more than enough pills. Perhaps we're here

today to keep the DEA in check and prevent them from taking any other drastic measures. The court order for the fine against Walgreens was signed by the Administrator of the DEA, Michele M. Leonhart. She is no longer with the DEA.

We also need to discuss the inaction by those who could put an end to this crisis. Our attorney general has referred to the high prescribing doctors as "drug dealers in white coats," but our BOM is not revoking their license. A pill mill/pain clinic could not operate without a doctor.

Medical Quality Assurance (MQA) License Verification:

Cynthia Cadet License Verification *8/10/2015

Discipline on File: No

Public complaint: Yes

License: Delinquent

Complaints on file: Seven

Case # 2009-15100: Four counts, one of which is: The quantities and/or combinations of controlled substances prescribed were inappropriate: signed by State Surgeon General H. Frank Farmer, December, 2011.

Case # 2010-08048: Fifteen counts, one of which is: The quantities and/or combinations of controlled substances prescribed were inappropriate: signed by State Surgeon General, April 2015.

Case # 2011-13720: The offense charged in Count 13 is otherwise commonly referred to as "money laundering": signed October 2014, State Surgeon General John H. Armstrong.

———

Paul Henry Wand License Verification *8/10/15

License: Clear/Active

Discipline on File: Yes

Public Complaint: Yes

Case # 2009-23424: The medical records obtained in response to the subpoena documented that Respondent had prescribed large amounts and doses of controlled substances to patients: CV, RD, LM, AC, DC, and RL: signed Surgeon General John H. Armstrong, September 2012.

The Florida Medical Association (FMA) could also help this crisis. STOPPNow is gathering support to make the Prescription Drug Monitoring Program (PDMP) mandatory for physicians to use. Twenty other states in our country have enacted this measure as law. Florida has not. One legislator-told me that we must get the approval of the FMA or they will not sponsor such a bill. I would like to publicly ask Mark Rubenstein of the FMA to approve and help gain support for the mandate. This is an epidemic, and every pill has been prescribed.

I did not have time for further explanation, as they notified me of my time limit. I would like to have explained that if the Board of Medicine would take the bad doctors out of the equation, there are plenty of pills for those who truly need them. I was able to question the distributor from Cardinal Health regarding my confusion as to the quotas he was mentioning of 5,000/month for a pharmacy. The DEA's Susan Langston had also been able to earlier state that the DEA does not put any quotas on a pharmacy. I stated that 5,000/month = 60,000 a year; these seem like such innocent numbers. I stated the list of court documents regarding pharmacies that had gone from 388,000 units of oxycodone a year to over two million a year was what caused the DEA to seek an indictment.

Many of the pharmacists spoke of their fear of losing their license if they fill prescriptions that should not have been filled. And they have no clear distinction. If a pharmacist sees a red flag, they are just telling the consumer they have no more pills. So this is another kink that must be worked out.

What was not spoken of is the greed that got us here. And I'm sorry I did not have time to tell them of a person who came to me and told of a family-owned pharmacy. It seems the son realized there was a golden opportunity for him to cash in. He was selling oxycodone – no prescription needed – to the neighborhood. And when a cancer patient came in who truly needed the pills, they were turned away.

I thought the meeting was very beneficial. Although the committee chair, Gavin Meshad, mentioned they are the Board of Pharmacy and are limited in what they can do, he is forming a workshop in Tallahassee to try to come up with some solutions. Nabil El Sanadi, M.D., Florida Board of Medicine, volunteered to be a member of the workshop.

FMA representative Mark Rubenstein said he would send someone. My last statement was to ask the FMA for their approval of mandating the PDMP. I did receive an affirmative nod of head, but when I spoke to Dr. Mark Rubenstein afterward, he stated that the FMA and the AMA, of which he is also a part, will only recommend that the doctors use the PDMP, not mandate it. His reasoning was that if a doctor didn't use it, he could go to jail. That, of course, is total nonsense.

Dr. Mark Rubinstein. You'll see his name again. I don't believe in coincidences.

CHAPTER FIFTEEN

Law Enforcement and DEA Is All We Have

A couple of years ago, when Vincent Coangello (Mr. $150,000 a day) was first arrested, the Federal Prosecutor sent me an email and asked that I get in touch with him. Very curious as to why a federal prosecutor would want to talk with me, I called him. It turned out that, since prescription drugs are legal, prosecuting the pill-mill owners and doctors hadn't been done too often. So, he wanted to make sure he could get a conviction. He needed information. I told him that I didn't want in any way to mislead him into thinking I knew more than I did. We know through word of mouth where the pain clinics are and stand outside with protest signs.

In the case of that particular pain clinic, a community civic association had called and asked us to come. The line in the morning waiting for the pain clinic to open would wrap around the building, the association told us. When I reported this, the prosecutor said he understood and the phone call ended.

A couple of months went by, and he called me again. I happened to be home sick from work. I had some kind of flu and was not feeling up to par. He initiated the conversation by saying he understood if I was afraid to talk. I responded, "No. You don't know me at all. If I knew anything, I would tell you." I wanted them arrested. I wanted them to quit killing for money. He asked if I would come down and see him, stating that he wanted to know what I know. He wanted to pick my brain. I agreed that when I was feeling better I would come down. I remember him asking, "Well, when do you think you'll be feeling better? Can you come down in two days?"

Renee (the mother with whom I formed STOPPNow) and I went downtown together. We were introduced to the prosecutor's team, who were all seated at a large table. One of the team members was a police detective who used to come out to our protests. He would always be in a discreet car, dressed in plain clothes, parked a parking lot away. The detective told me I should not draw any attention to the fact that I was there. I would bring over any mother who had empty pill bottles with doctors' names on them to share with him.

The meeting lasted several hours, much longer than we anticipated. We shared our stories; the team members shared theirs. The federal prosecutor had a multitude of files they had confiscated during the raid of Vincent Coangello's pill mill. He told us something that we didn't know: Renee's son, Blayne, was in the file. Blayne had visited the pain clinic the day before he walked in front of the car on State Road 7 and was killed.

I gave the prosecutor another name to check. There is another mother and father suffering the loss of their child. Her friend sends me a donation every year on Jon's birthday and another on the anniversary of his death. Jon's name was not in the file. We were pretty certain that it was Joel Shumrak's pain clinic that helped him to lose his life. Those records went to Kentucky. I was not able to get them for the mother.

It is hard to get a prosecution against a doctor. Blayne walked in front of a car on a six-lane highway. Jon was in a car accident. The question still remains why these "drug dealer doctors" are able to keep their licensure. That is the Board of Medicine's job: to protect the public. These were good kids before this drug destroyed their lives and, of course, those of their parents.

When STOPPNow first started, there were no consequences to either clinic owners or doctors. Then they started arresting some doctors for money laundering and tax evasion. Then some clinic owners began to be arrested. Finally, in 2011, Dr. Gerald Klein was charged with first-degree murder for the death of Joseph Bartolucci.

CHAPTER SIXTEEN

First Degree Murder Charge: State vs. Dr. Gerald J. Klein

When STOPPNow first started protesting outside of pill mills, the doctors and pill-mill owners on the inside consistently escaped responsibility for the deaths related to the massive distribution of drugs issuing from these "clinics" because, technically, the clinics were not breaking the law. Oxycodone, Xanax, and Soma, the drugs most often dispensed from these establishments, are all legal prescription drugs. Finally, however, the system has begun to hold those on the inside accountable for their actions. Dr. Cynthia Cadet and Dr. Gerald Klein, among others, have been called to answer for their connection to the pill-mill industry.

Dr. Cadet and Dr. Klein were both hired to write prescriptions for twin brothers Chris and Jeffrey (Jeff) George's pill mills. (The George brothers, who built a pill-mill empire, are just two of many players in Florida's tragic prescription-pill situation. One of Jeff George's clinics, East Coast Pain Clinic, was the setting for the activities resulting in the charges against Dr. Gerald Klein.)

Dr. Cadet went to trial before Dr. Klein. Although she was charged with contributing to the death of six people, ultimately, Dr. Cadet was convicted only of money laundering. I was concerned about the outcome of Dr. Cadet's trial, so when I became aware of Dr. Klein's trial, I was determined to make the one-hour trip to the West Palm Beach Court every day and record what I saw and heard.

Dr. Klein's three-week trial began on Monday, August 24, 2015, and concluded on Tuesday, September 15, 2015. I attended the trial starting on Trial Day Four: Thursday, August 27, 2015. Having missed Days One through Three, I also missed Jeff George's testimony. But for years I have followed accounts of his and his brother's unpunished acts, their lack of accountability, and their disregard of the deaths caused by their businesses. In fact, STOPPNow protested outside of more than one pain clinic owned by the George brothers. However, once they realized we weren't going away, they started to close the clinics on the days our protests were scheduled. We had rattled their nerves.

Starting on Trial Day Four: Thursday, August 27, 2015, I sat in the courtroom of the West Palm Beach Courthouse and took detailed notes. The transcript of the trial that follows is excerpted from my own personal notes, made during the hours I spent watching the trial unfold. However, provided there have been no court orders to seal or expunge the records, the full, official court transcripts are available to the public at www.mypalmbeachclerk.com.

Before we delve into my notes, let me orient you to the basic charges and participants:

Dr. Gerald Klein was charged with first-degree murder as the result of the death of twenty-four-year-old Joseph Bartolucci, who frequented the pill mill known as East Coast Pain Clinic, 6706 Okeechobee Boulevard, Suites 53 and 54, West Palm Beach, Florida, owned by Jeff George. As an agent of East Coast Pain Clinic, Dr. Klein wrote prescriptions for Oxycodone, Xanax, and Soma—the cocktail of drugs that East Coast Pain, like other pill mills, dispensed on a cash-only basis. (Before the trial even started, the defense team successfully convinced the judge to forbid the use of the phrase "pill mill" during the trial.)

In Broward County, the epicenter of the pill-mill epidemic, instances of doctors meeting clients in motel rooms, doctors connecting with patients in Starbucks, and doctors exchanging pills for sexual favors have all been documented. There are also, no doubt, decent men, like Gerald Klein seems to me to be, who succumb to the temptation of greed. In Dr. Klein's case, this temptation led to him sitting in a courthouse, charged with first-degree murder.

Circuit Court Judge Karen Miller presided over Dr. Klein's murder trial. I found her to be fair and to demonstrate a no-nonsense attitude toward the proceedings in her courtroom.

Assistant State Attorney Barbara Burns represented the State as the lead prosecutor in the case. She seemed to be a gentle person. She sometimes appeared flustered when looking through her files for a needed document.

Assistant State Attorney Mike Rachel was the second chair for the prosecution of Dr. Klein.

Defense Attorney Sam Rabin represented Dr. Klein. As a defense attorney, he was bold, intimidating, and appeared to be furious towards witnesses at times. Even when Attorney Rabin kept the court waiting while he looked through his files, he still seemed aggressive. As a result, it seemed, no mention of his being unprepared was ever expressed.

Defense Attorney Michael R. Band was the second chair on the defense team for Dr. Klein.

DAY FOUR: THURSDAY, AUGUST 27, 2015

THE STATE CALLS: THEODORE OBERMEYER

Theodore Obermeyer (sometimes referred to in these notes as "Theo") doesn't appear to be someone who would end up in prison. He once had a contractor's license and was able to provide a stable income for his family. That is, until the housing bubble burst. When construction jobs evaporated, though, his old neighborhood friends the George brothers were only too happy to oblige him with a new career. Chris and Jeff George were making millions. Jeff George offered Obermeyer a job managing one of his pill mills, although Theo's new job managing the day-to-day operation of the pill mill was not as lucrative for him as it was for Jeff George.

An investigation found that "The brothers' clinics were thriving like never before in early 2010, having made nearly $1 million dollars in a single week in late February. But on the morning of March 3, they were awakened by urgent phone calls. The clinics were being raided by the DEA task force" (Investigations, NBC NEWS, 2012).

Theo is serving time, now, away from his family, for making a very bad decision.

> PROSECUTOR BARBARA BURNS: Mr. Obermeyer can you tell the court where you reside?
>
> OBERMEYER: Yes. The Federal Corrections Institute in Miami. I pleaded guilty to trafficking oxycodone.
>
> Q. And your sentence?
>
> A. 144 months.
>
> Q. And you were charged by federal court?
>
> A. Yes.
>
> Q. And you have agreed to testify for the state?
>
> A. Yes.
>
> Q. Maximum penalty for the State charge of second-degree murder is twenty years. Do you have any medical training?
>
> A. No, ma'am.
>
> Q. How do you know Jeffrey George?
>
> A. We have been friends since we were three years old.
>
> Q. And where have you been employed?
>
> A. I worked as area manager for Jeffrey George's father's construction business. The business failed. I then worked for Jeff George's Health and Wellness Clinic, doing phone sales for steroids. Two to three months.

Then Jeff George asked me to do some remodeling on a building in a strip mall that he was going to use as a medical clinic. He needed to have a doctor's exam room, a pharmacy in back, and a waiting room. When I was through with the construction, Jeff asked me to manage the chronic pain facility.

Q. Have you ever worked with chronic pain?

A. No.

Q. Any education to manage a clinic?

A. No.

Q. Did Jeff George have any medical training?

A. No.

Q. How much were you paid as the manager?

A. $1,500 a week.

Q. When did the pain clinic open?

A. Around the spring of 2008.

Q. How did you advertise for medical staff?

A. Craigslist, HeadHunters.

Q. So, somewhere around the spring of 2008, when you opened, the employees included yourself and Jeff George. Anyone else?

A. Yes. Ally Ruiz.

Q. A CV [*curriculum vitae*] was received from Dr. Gerald Klein before the opening. Did you and Jeff George interview Dr. Klein?

A. Yes.

Q. What were the topics?

A. Medications prescribed, background, type of facility he worked for. He had been an army doctor and surgeon. He was currently working at a pain management office in Boynton Beach.

Q. Was the type of medication discussed?

A. I had no knowledge, but discussion was about oxycodone 30 mg and Xanax 2 mg. Jeff asked what he was prescribing and was he in agreement with the amount 180-240.

Q. Did Dr. Klein say anything?

A. He said every patient was different, but that he was familiar with those doses.

Q. Were they both in agreement?

DEFENSE ATTORNEY: Objection. Leading.

PROSECUTOR: Did Dr. Klein say he was in agreement with the amount of 180-240 pills?

OBERMEYER: Yes. Dr. Klein said he wanted to work part time, three days a week.

Q. When the clinic first opened, was Dr. Klein the only doctor employed?

A. Yes.

Q. What hours were you open?

A. Monday through Friday, 9-5. Then two to three months later, we hired a second doctor.

Q. What kind of paperwork did the business have?

A. We had a patient sign-in sheet, in-house pharmacy license and rules. Jeff had all the paperwork and forms. He made sure that the doctors had a dispensing license. Once the clinic had a doctor's DEA license on file, I was able to start ordering medications.

Q. How did you know how much to order?

A. Jeff said max out what they'll allow. A 2-2-2 form was needed for ordering. [DEA Controlled Substance Order Form DEA 222]

Q. Can you sign the form?

A. No, a doctor's signature is required. The doctor that signed was Dr. Klein.

Q. Was there any discussion about the quantity?

A. No.

Q. Any discussion about there being so many wholesalers?

A. No.

Q. Who signed for the medications when they were delivered?

A. Dr. Klein.

Q. How were the doctors paid?

A. Starting salary was $150 an hour.

Q. Did you advertise?

A. We used the Internet, newspapers, pay-per-click, Google "back pain," "neck pain." Advertisers pay for their pain clinics to pop up. The clinic paid every time someone clicked on.

Q. Were the newspapers mainstream?

A. No, underground. *New Times*, and so forth. Circulation was in strip malls, strip clubs.

Q. Any discounts?

A. Yes. The special was $100 for a first-time visit.

Q. Did you take insurance?

A. No.

Q. Did you take cash or credit cards?

A. Yes. We did not accept insurance for the in-house pharmacy either.

Q. Were there ever any meetings regarding a patient's sickness?

A. No.

Q. What did the exam rooms look like? Did they have an exam table, blood pressure cuff, desk, sink?

A. No sink.

Q. Gloves?

A. Yes.

Q. Paper for the table?

A. No.

Q. Was there ever any discussion to not do things to attract attention?

A. Yes. Out of state patients drew attention and seeing clients under the age of twenty-five.

Q. When Dr. Klein had concerns, did you and Jeff George agree not to see patients under twenty-five?

A. Yes.

Q. Did you see patients under twenty-five?

A. Yes.

Q. How did you determine if the patients were out of state or not?

A. They provided a phone or electric bill.

Q. Did Dr. Klein still see patients from out of state? Did Dr. Klein express concern about undercover agents?

A. Yes.

DEFENSE: Objection.

PROSECUTOR: What was Dr. Klein's concern?

DEFENSE: Objection.

JUDGE: Witness may answer.

OBERMEYER: Dr. Klein wanted to make sure that the information filed, that we must dot all the i's and cross all the t's.

PROSECUTOR: Was that said to do everything right or appearance?

DEFENSE: Objection.

A break for lunch was called. After the jury was excused, the judge and the two lead attorneys discussed issues that each side had—among them, the inclusion of East Coast Pain Clinic patient logs as evidence. The prosecutor wanted to show that the number of patients seen on any given day exceeded the number provided for by "standard of care." The patient logs also document the amounts of cash a client would walk in with to pay for their visit and purchase pills. (So-called patients walking into a so-called doctor's office with thousands of dollars in cash in their pockets to purchase drugs!)

The defense argued that the prosecution was trying to prejudice the jury because the patient logs showed that all patients were given the same number of pills all day, every day. The defense also made the point that the jury should not be allowed to see patients' medical records, as doing so would be a HIPAA (Health Insurance Portability and Accountability Act of 1996) violation. However, the names of those patients not involved in the case had been blacked out in accordance with HIPAA.

We have all heard accounts of a jury rendering a not-guilty verdict due to the prosecution's inability to show evidence they needed to convict. During the weeks I spent in the West Palm Beach courtroom, I learned that the evidence may well be available, but if the defense team is successful in getting the judge to disallow it, it will not be introduced to the jury.

In this case, however, the judge ruled the patient logs and cash logs (also referred to as "customer data logs" during the trial) admissible, and the jury was called back in and proceedings resumed.

> PROSECUTOR: One hundred percent of your patients got narcotics. Yet, the answer to the question on the form was that sixty to seventy percent of patients being seen are receiving narcotics. Did Dr. Klein have to sign that form?
>
> OBERMEYER: I'm not one hundred percent sure.
>
> Q. Do you recall if the forms required a DEA number? And then a doctor would have to sign off on it?

A. Yes.

Q. Did Dr. Klein ever complain that the information on the form was not accurate?

A. No.

Q. Who would dispense at the in-house pharmacy?

A. Myself or Ally Ruiz would.

Q. Did the doctor observe?

A. No.

Q. Did the doctor sign off after each prescription?

A. No. At the end of the day he would sign off on the list.

Q. Were you or Ms. Ruiz registered pharmacists?

A. No.

Q. How often was Jeff George at the clinic?

A. Maybe six or seven times since the opening. We talked every day. I would report to him regarding how many patients were seen each day. Copies of the daily logs were faxed, along with the daily cash log and the daily prescription log.

Q. Did you ever receive patient complaints?

A. Yes. Jeff George would call and tell me when a patient called him to complain about the number of pills they had been prescribed. I would then speak to the doctors to make sure the patients were happy. From opening to March, there were only a handful of complaints. I had a conversation with Dr. Klein that Jeff received a complaint about a decrease in the amount of pills. I would tell him this is a business, and Dr. Klein agreed to increase.

Q. Let's say a patient was receiving a prescription for 240 pills, and the new script was for 210. Did he change the prescription?

A. Yes.

Q. Did you make it clear to Dr. Klein that Jeff George wanted to make sure the patients were happy? Happy with the medication they received? Did Jeff George speak to you regarding what to do about a doctor who refused?

A. None refused.

Q. Were alternate methods of treatment other than narcotics ever offered to patients?

A. No.

Q. Were patients encouraged to use the in-house pharmacy?

A. Yes. They were told that it was easier than going to Walgreens.

Q. The clinic was shut down March 3, 2010. Were there any other doctors who were there the whole time?

A. No. Just Dr. Klein.

Q. Were steps taken to make East Coast Pain Clinic appear legitimate?

A. Papers were filled out by Jeff George and Dr. Klein. I filed them, but did not know what they meant.

Q. Who was responsible for the daily deposits?

A. I was. I would count the money and fax a copy to Jeff and then make the deposit.

Q. Were any drugs diverted from the in-house pharmacy?

A. Yes.

Q. By whom?

A. I knew Jeff took pills. I don't know what he did with them.

Q. What did you do?

A. One time I took 2,400 pills. I sold them for $12,000, just the one time. I also gave Jeff Xanax for his wife one time. When Jeff took pills, he adjusted the numbers in the computer, the inventory.

Q. Did you become aware there was an oxycodone shortage in 2009?

A. Yes. I told Jeff, then Dr. Klein.

Q. What medication was the biggest income for the clinic?

A. Oxycodone. The solution by Dr. Klein was that we could use hydromorphone. There was a nationwide shortage of oxycodone. I called every distributor from California to New York to find another distributor that had it in stock.

Q. Did you finally order hydromorphone?

A. Yes.

Q. What milligram?

A. 4 mg. Dr. Klein had said that the drug came in 4 mg and 8 mg, but comparable order 4 mg.

Q. Was the order placed for 4 mg and signed off by Dr. Klein?

A. Yes.

Q. Did the doctors prescribe hydromorphone?

A. Yes, at 4 mg.

Q. Do you remember how long?

A. Roughly two months.

Q. There was a question as to whether the file of the deceased had been altered.

DEFENSE: Objection.

All approached the bench. Many times during the trial, reference was made to Dr. Klein's handwriting being illegible.

PROSECUTOR: There are documents in the file dated December 12, 2008, another document dated January 20, 2009, and another document February 27, 2009. There is no explanation of how they got into the file. The notes appear to be typed notes of the assessment. Do you know anything about these?

OBERMEYER: There was a meeting regarding the death of Joseph Bartolucci behind closed doors. Jeff George, Dr. Klein, and a lawyer were in attendance. After the death, business was back to normal at the clinic.

PROSECUTOR: How much in revenue would the pain clinic take in on a normal day?

DEFENSE: Objection.

All to the bench.

PROSECUTOR: Do you know what Dr. Klein earned per week?

OBERMEYER: $4,200 per week.

Not bad for three days a week. It is now 4:50 p.m., and the trial closes for the day. The defense will begin questioning the same witness, Theodore Obermeyer, tomorrow.

DAY FIVE: FRIDAY, AUGUST 28, 2015

DEFENSE: SAME WITNESS, THEODORE OBERMEYER

DEFENSE: You're here today because you want to reduce your sentence.

Throughout the trial, the defense attorney was noted for making statements rather than asking questions. Sometimes the witnesses could barely get their answers in.

OBERMEYER: I want the court to know the truth.

DEFENSE: You could not lower your sentence without passing through this court. Isn't that right?

A. Yes.

Q. 144 months. A twelve-year sentence. You pleaded guilty in order to get a reduction. Federal Court Rule 35.

The defense attorney is referring to a Rule 35 motion, which is a motion filed by a prosecutor under the authority granted by the Federal Rules of Criminal Procedure. It asks a court to reduce a previously imposed sentence based on "substantial assistance" by a defendant, provided after sentencing.

DEFENSE: Only a federal court can make that change. Originally, with the federal sentence, you could have been facing seventy years.

OBERMEYER: Yes.

Q. Your attorney was able to eliminate three counts if you pleaded guilty to one count, max twenty years. The judge gave you twelve years because you are cooperating. This was due to Rule 35. Now, back to the first question. You are here today because you have to cooperate and be here. Part of the deal to cooperate with the State was they took information from you. Whatever information you had. Then they sucker punched you, didn't they?

PROSECUTOR: Objection.

DEFENSE: They got the information that they needed, then they told you that you would be charged with second degree murder. You didn't have any feeling that you had any role in the murder, did you? You didn't even know he visited East Coast Pain?

OBERMEYER: No. I knew he visited East Coast Pain. I didn't know how many times.

Q. It was at a deposition with Prosecutor Burns where you said you didn't know the patient. Like I said, defense gets a copy of the deposition and reads it. At first you didn't recognize the name. You knew you had to plead guilty to testify. You're now moved from federal prison. They moved you to West Palm Beach.

A. Yes.

Q. You are currently on Gun Club Road, with Chris Hutson.

A. Yes.

Q. Isn't he a defendant with you?

A. Yes.

Q. Isn't that a violation of your agreement, to be with Chris Hutson on Gun Club Road?

PROSECUTOR: Objection.

Both attorneys approach the bench. Questioning resumes.

DEFENSE: They have an open-door pod. You and he are friends.

OBERMEYER: I wouldn't call us friends.

Q. You cannot have any contact with a co-witness.

A. Unfortunately, I have no choice where they put me.

Q. You could have asked as part of your plea agreement to be moved.

A. I haven't read my plea agreement in four years.

Q. Let me show you what you signed. So, in other words, you could go back and talk about the case.

A. If I wanted to.

Q. You didn't try to get moved.

A. I didn't know I could, at the time.

Q. Do you know why they keep witnesses separate? We have established that you had to testify. You thought you were being charged with trafficking. You thought it was Xanax. You could have been charged with first-degree murder. It was due to a plea that you were charged with second-degree murder. First-degree murder would have been an automatic life in prison. Second count punishable by thirty years but cap twenty. But if you cooperate, the cap goes away. The twenty-year cap. No minimum, fifteen years.

A. Yes.

Q. If you don't cooperate, Ms. Burns won't work with you.

A. I just know I'm facing twenty years.

Q. The federal charge is concurrent with the state, and the state is concurrent with federal. You know this is going to help you.

A. Yes.

Q. You shake your head, but you know. OK. So after leaving Jeff George's father's employ you worked at SE Rejuvenate [steroids]. You quit because you weren't comfortable, not sure if it was legal, right?

A. Yes.

Q. You have a contractor's license. You're a smart guy. Then George has you construct his building. Then George says, "We're friends. Come to my pain clinic." Did you know he owned other clinics?

A. I only knew about one.

Q. Did you say to Jeff, "I don't want to get involved if it's illegal"?

A. Yes.

Q. Then Jeff said, "Theo, I have done everything legal. I have lawyers." He led you to believe.... You knew about South Florida Pain. He owned that with his brother. He told you about the laws and regulations. From the time you worked there until the end, you thought it was legit.

A. Towards the end, I had my doubts.

Q. Yeah, when you stole meds from Dr. Klein, you knew that wasn't legit. What did he expect of you?

A. I was going to oversee the transactions. Make sure that no one was stealing, monitor the doctors' time.

Q. Did he tell you the forms were reviewed by a lawyer?

A. Yes.

Q. So you felt comfortable?

A. Yes.

Q. Dr. Klein was hired through HeadHunters, not Craigslist.

A. They advertised on both, so I didn't know.

Q. He was used to pain patients. Oxycodone, Xanax, Percocet. I believe Dr. Klein said every patient is a different range, from 180-240. It was not dictated by George how much he would prescribe. Dr. Klein said "I can't give you specifics."

A. Yes.

Q. Dr. Klein said, "I want to work at a legitimate clinic," right?

A. Yes.

Q. Do you remember being cut off by the investigator when you said Dr. Klein said he wanted to work a long time at a reputable clinic?

A. Not that I recall.

Q. Here's the document.

A. It appears that I did stop.

Q. So, when you said something favorable about Dr. Klein, you were cut off. Dr. Klein said he wanted $100 an hour. That was the market at the time.

A. Yes.

Q. One raise from $150 to $180 an hour.

A. Yes. Jeff did the numbers.

Q. Dr. Klein was always hourly.

A. Yes.

Q. No lines outside.

A. No.

Q. Let's talk about the exam room. Yesterday, the prosecutor said that there were no sinks. But every exam room had Purell didn't they? Dr. Klein wanted MRI's.

A. Jeff and Dr. Klein wanted them.

Q. Didn't Dr. Klein want MRI's?

A. Yes.

Q. MRI's are something you took seriously.

A. Yes.

Q. You had a policy to review all MRI's.

A. Yes.

Q. You didn't know Jeff George was setting up fake MRI's.

A. No.

Personally, I like Theo, but I'm not sure if I believe him on this. A detective told me he was once called at 2:00 a.m. to a strip club. In the alley behind the club there was a mobile MRI unit. A long line of patrons was waiting to pay a fee to obtain an MRI.

DEFENSE: Dr. Klein trusted you with the inventory, and you were stealing from him.

OBERMEYER: Yes.

Q. You told the prosecutor yesterday that you had no experience in pain.

A. Yes.

Q. Let's discuss discharging patients. Dr. Klein discharged patients for a number of reasons.

A. The clinic and Dr. Klein.

Q. Let's talk about Dr. Klein. Did he discharge patients? For what reasons?

A. Doctor shopping [when a person goes to more than one doctor to get pills], IV drug use.

Q. What about failed drug test?

A. Sometimes.

Q. Did he review them all?

A. No.

While the jury went to lunch, the defense moved to exclude the testimony of Chris Hutson, due to his proximity to Obermeyer while in detention, stating that Chris Hutson and Theo Obermeyer could talk about events of the trial. The prosecutor rebutted, saying that the witnesses were never asked if they discussed the case, and that she could certainly develop that conversation in front of the jury. The defense said that, in fact, he was being asked to take whatever answer the witness gave him, and that is why there is a rule. (For once, I can understand the defense attorney's argument.) Without the jury present, the defense questioned Obermeyer.

DEFENSE: Tell us what you have discussed. First of all, did you discuss the upcoming trial? Talk about when the case is over? Will Chris Hutson be getting out? You talked about general things. Did you talk about what you are going to testify?

OBERMEYER: No.

DEFENSE: Does Chris Hutson have any of his depositions with him?

OBERMEYER: I don't know.

DEFENSE: Do you?

OBERMEYER: No.

Jury back. Court in session.

DEFENSE: Let's discuss the in-house pharmacy. You told the jury that Dr. Klein had very little to do with setting up the pharmacy. When, in fact, Dr. Klein did discuss storing the inventory?

OBERMEYER: That was after it was setup.

Q. You knew that Dr. Klein relied on you to run the pharmacy. You took the inventory to Dr. Klein every day.

A. Yes.

Q. You did full inventories. You would prepare the document and bring it to Dr. Klein to sign.

A. I would take a daily inventory, then hand count what was in the safe.

Q. You had a system that labeled and kept track of the meds. You had a sophisticated system. It tracked inventory control, patient ID, accounts receivable, bar codes. In fact, major pharmacies use this system. You learned how to use it.

A. Yes.

Q. You never told him that you were stealing.

A. No.

Q. You testified that you had no pharmacy credentials.

A. Yes.

Q. Ms. Ruiz did have tech training.

A. She was trained on how to use the inventory system.

Q. There was a certificate that hung in the pharmacy. Person certified to dispense.

A. Yes.

Q. Certifying Dispensing Tech.

A. She received that from training on the inventory system.

Q. You told the jury that you diverted drugs two times.

A. I did it twice.

Q. Explain that.

A. The second one I gave directly to Jeff for his wife.

Q. You never expected to be charged by the state.

A. Correct.

Q. How many pills?

A. 2,400.

Q. You never told Dr. Klein because you didn't want him to know you were doing anything illegal. You didn't want to lie to him.

A. Correct.

Q. Your basis of knowledge was from Dr. Klein and Jeff.

A. Yes.

Q. Patients at East Coast Pain generally had a diagnosis.

A. Not for me to say.

Q. These were people who had documented injuries. That was most of your patients, right?

A. Yes.

Q. You had dozens of complaints of Dr. Klein cutting back on medications. You went to Dr. Klein. He would say to you, "If there is enough information, I will try to go back up."

A. Sometimes we would compromise.

Q. He said he would only do it if comfortable. Dr. Klein would say, "I'll only adjust the amount if I'm comfortable doing it," correct?

A. Yes.

Q. You said in the interview that Dr. Klein said range from 180-240. Here is the document of Dr. Klein's CV. There is writing on the side next to the Roxies, and there is a line drawn to 180, with 240 being crossed out. Do you know why?

A. I remember him saying that he's not comfortable writing more than 240.

Q. You were interviewed by the DEA how many times?

A. I think four.

Q. After that you met with Ms. Burns. How many times?

A. About six or seven.

Q. How many interviews on the federal side?

A. Maybe one or two.

Q. The deposition was taken in February. How many times after the deposition did you meet with DEA, FBI?

A. None besides the seven.

Q. What about the federal prosecutor?

A. Probably three.

Q. Did the prosecutor tell you what questions she was going to ask you?

A. Yes.

Q. Did she tell you what I was going to say?

A. No, she didn't. She didn't coach me.

Q. Now, the DEA interviews. You told the agent that his scripts were 100-210 range. That's a lot lower than 180. Do you remember how much Joseph Bartolucci received on his first visit?

A. 150.

Q. Below 180, right?

A. Yes.

Q. Do you remember the second prescription?

A. Which med?

Q. Oxycodone.

A. 150.

Q. That was the first time. What about the second time?

A. 180.

Q. Back to the document. [Shows it to Obermeyer] Does that refresh your memory?

A. 120.

Q. OK. That went down. First time, 150. Would you accept 15 mg?

A. If that's what the file said.

Q. Second time, 30 mg. That being said, you would have to know what happened with the patient. Was he getting pain relief?

The quantity went from 150 to 120, but the dosage was 15 mg oxycodone on the first visit, and Dr. Klein prescribed 30 mg of oxycodone on the second visit. That dosage is double the amount of the earlier dosage. That is not a decrease. Of course, the jury heard the defense attorney say it was a decrease, and that is probably what will stick with them.

OBERMEYER: Yes.

DEFENSE: You know that the people coming to East Coast had chronic pain?

PROSECUTOR: Objection.

DEFENSE: They said they had chronic pain.

OBERMEYER Yes.

Q. What's Suboxone?

This is a drug that can help when a patient is trying to withdraw. It can also be abused.

OBERMEYER: It's a drug that replaces the opiate.

DEFENSE: Is it your understanding that the same doctor that prescribes for pain can also prescribe this?

A. Yes. You have to be certified.

Q. Dr. Klein said in his interview that he wanted to treat with Suboxone. Dr. Klein told you he wanted to offer Suboxone.

A. Yes.

Q. Now, this was not the business model you and Jeff discussed.

A. Yes. But anything that made money.

Q. I'm not asking you that. Dr. Klein didn't want to see patients under-twenty-five or out of state.

A. Correct.

Q. Dr. Klein said that he didn't want to treat anyone under the age of twenty-five, unless it was an extreme case. Then, in respect to out of state patients, he said these are potential problems.

A. Yes.

Q. Do you remember when the shortage of oxycodone occurred?

A. The best evidence of the date would be when the clinic started prescribing Dilaudid, due to the DEA production limit.

Pills were being dispensed like it was a candy store. The DEA is still being blamed for the production quotas. Meanwhile, every year, the death rate from prescription-drug poisoning increases. The drug companies that produce these highly addictive drugs maintain the ability to keep them in the marketplace.

DEFENSE: Either way, you still had patients who had pain or claimed to have pain. Dr. Klein researched to find out how to help the patients. He called other people, got on the Internet. What he found was Dilaudid. There are formulations, tables on how to figure out the conversion amount. Calculations that he rechecked after [Joseph Bartolucci's] death. Do you remember saying 30 mg oxycodone equals 4 mg of Dilaudid? How did you come up with that?

OBERMEYER: On the Internet.

Q. You were coming in and out of the meeting.

A. No.

Q. Do you recall Dr. Klein asking the office staff during that meeting to type up his notes?

A. No, I don't.

Q. You had a conversation with Dr. Klein after the death. He said [Joseph Bartolucci] was a good kid; he felt bad about the death. You could tell he was depressed at work after that. Dr. Klein would give you cards for files to refer people out.

A. I believe he wrote them on prescriptions.

Q. You knew that Jeff George was involved in bad things. Shooting out windows of competitors, kidnapping. You stayed away from that.

A. Yes.

Q. You testified that East Coast Pain Clinic had no other modality of treatment, but in fact Dr. Klein did. Yesterday, you stated that you never had to threaten doctors. In fact, you did say, "If you don't see patients faster, we'll fire you."

A. Yes.

Q. On the Bartolucci file that the prosecutor showed you yesterday, at the time you pleaded guilty to second-degree murder. You were able to leave on bond.

A. Yes.

Q. Jeff George offered you $50,000 to leave the country.

A. Yes.

Q. You didn't go.

A. No.

Q. Do you feel Jeff George used you?

A. Yes.

PROSECUTOR: ON REDIRECT, THEODORE OBERMEYER

PROSECUTOR: Were you willing to stay after you learned that the business was not legitimate?

OBERMEYER: I guess you could say I was in too deep by then.

Q. Did the money and benefits factor into your decision?

A. Yes.

PROSECUTOR: No more questions for this witness, Your Honor.

THE STATE CALLS: MS. ALLY RUIZ

Ally Ruiz is a young woman in her early twenties. She is clearly petrified to be here. She explains that she has a young daughter and was glad to find a job on Craigslist that allowed her to have weekends off and normal office hours. This arrangement enabled her to care for her baby. She is a likable girl and obviously didn't know what she had signed up for.

She worked at the front desk at East Coast Pain Clinic signing patients in and collecting cash for payment—and sometimes filling the pharmacy orders. Her testimony is important because it enables the prosecutor to introduce the customer data log, mentioned previously (also referred to as patient log). With the names of the patients blacked out, the evidence will be used only to reveal the amounts of cash being paid. Since Ally Ruiz is familiar with the contents of the patient log, she can explain it to the jury. (As mentioned earlier, the defense argued to keep the log out, stating that it was a HIPAA violation. "HIPAA violation," however, has become a catch phrase to keep much needed legislation from being introduced or passed into law. HIPAA violation was cited in Florida, when there was great opposition to passing the PDMP—which did pass into law in 2011. However, there was no patient violation then, and there is no patient violation here.)

> PROSECUTOR: Ms. Ruiz, you were an employee of East Coast Pain Clinic. You have no medical experience?
>
> MS. RUIZ: No. I found an ad on Craigslist. Front desk, no weekends. I interviewed with Chris Hutson at SE Rejuvenation. It was behind a strip club. I was there three or four months.
>
> Q. Did you ever find out they were selling steroids?
>
> DEFENSE: Objection.
>
> PROSECUTOR: So you were there four months, and you didn't know what they were doing.

MS. RUIZ: Mr. Hutson told me he was going to try to get me a job at a doctor's office, East Coast Pain Clinic.

Q. When you started there, do you recall who was the only doctor there?

A. Dr. Klein.

Q. How long did you stay at East Coast Pain Clinic?

A. Until the whole thing happened.

Q. The DEA raid?

A. Yes.

Q. Was Dr. Klein there the whole time?

A. Yes.

Q. Do you remember Dr. Jones?

A. I know he was one of the newer doctors. He was there about six months.

Q. Did you have any medical assistants?

A. No.

Q. Any registered nurses?

A. No. Theo trained me.

Q. How were you paid?

A. Cash at first, then check. About $700 a week.

Q. When you were working there, did anyone try to tip you?

A. Yes, if they wanted to get to the front of the line.

Q. Let's focus on the people coming in. Were any of them from out of state?

A. I believe for a short time.

Q. You became aware that people were driving the entire state of Florida to get to East Coast Pain Clinic. When was it decided you wouldn't see them anymore? Do you know if Dr. Klein saw out of state patients?

A. Yes.

Q. Did he ever indicate that he didn't want to see any out of state patients?

A. Yes.

Q. How many people would come in to see Dr. Klein?

DEFENSE: Objection.

PROSECUTOR: Did they have to have cash to see a doctor?

MS. RUIZ: Yes. They paid first.

Q. Do you recall how much they had to pay?

A. If they had a coupon, $50. With no coupon $150 to $200.

Q. Do you remember how much for a follow-up visit?

A. $150.

The prosecutor holds the customer data log for Ally to read and explain to the jury as she asks questions relating to the context. The log under consideration is the customer data log for February 2, 2009.

PROSECUTION: This column would be for the drugs they received. How about insurance?

MS. RUIZ: We did not take insurance.

Q. The first line in the total column is $594. So you would have people walking in that door with over $500 in cash?

A. Yes.

Q. Did that concern you?

A. Not at the time.

Q. Everyone who came to the clinic would have to sign in to this page if they were to be seen?

A. Yes.

Q. [pointing] This one here came in with $1,000?

DEFENSE: Objection.

PROSECUTOR: So, continuing, $1,000 would reflect what this customer paid?

MS. RUIZ: Yes.

Q. Who was involved after the person came out of the room with the doctor? Did you ever dispense drugs?

A. Sometimes I would.

Q. Who would handle putting pills in the bottle and taking cash?

A. They would have to pay first.

Q. Where was it kept?

A. At the front desk.

Q. Did you sometimes find shortages?

A. Yes.

Q. Sometimes 1,000 pills missing?

A. Yes.

Q. Did you ever bring this up to Theo?

A. Yes.

Q. What would he say?

A. "Are you sure you did the count right?" He would say I must have made a mistake.

Q. Were you ever told to identify with initials even if it was not checked?

A. Yes. I was told to hurry up, just initial that it's verified. Very rushed. The patients were waiting sometimes hours.

Q. Do you recall within the office when [Joseph Bartolucci's] death was discovered?

A. Yes. I don't think it was right away. I don't remember if it was Theo or Dr. Klein. But Dr. Klein wanted the file, and I gave it to him.

Q. Can you tell the jury how these three papers got on the chart?

They are referring to the medical records of the deceased, Joseph Bartolucci. A question was raised earlier as to whether or not the file had been altered after his death.

MS. RUIZ: I believe Theo asked me to stay late one night and sit with Dr. Klein to go over the patient's chart and type it for him. Dr. Klein sat next to me and told me what it said, and I typed it.

PROSECUTOR: You were typing what Dr. Klein was telling you?

A. Yes.

Q. So this is one of the notes, and you yourself couldn't read it. No insurance, no job, pain unchanged, epidural injection. Did the epidural injection ever occur?

A. No.

Q. Was there any other therapy offered?

A. No.

PROSECUTOR: No further questions, Your Honor.

DEFENSE: SAME WITNESS, ALLY RUIZ

DEFENSE: For a short period of time you accepted out of state patients. How long?

MS. RUIZ: A few months.

Q. How were you informed?

A. Theo.

Q. So out of state patients, whether they drove, flew, or horseback rode, they were not seen anymore. You had a policy that if somebody gave you an MRI you would verify it?

A. Most of the time.

Q. You said sometimes you were too rushed; then you would go back, right?

A. No, I would do it immediately.

Q. But it's clear that there was a policy to verify. You thought the clinic was legit, right? If you thought it was illegal, you would have left, right?

A. If I would have known this was going to be the outcome, I would have left, yes.

The prosecution asked a few questions on redirect, and then testimony for Day Five ended. Due to Hurricane Erika threatening South Florida, the West Palm Beach Courthouse was closed on Monday, August 31. The trial resumed on Tuesday, September 1.

DAY SIX: TUESDAY, SEPTEMBER 1, 2015

I've noticed a woman who comes into the courtroom occasionally and sits at the very end of a row, towards the back. She looks familiar, so once I was back home, I dug through my newspaper clippings and found her picture. She is Gina Bartolucci, Joseph Bartolucci's mother. The clipping I found is from February 2011, when I attended a memorial mass at Holy Name of Jesus Catholic Church. The mass, which was dedicated to overdose victims, was organized by Ms. Bartolucci and another mother who lost her son to prescription pills. Under Ms. Bartolucci's picture in the paper is a quote, which reads, *The mass is to honor those who died and those who have been left behind.*

Ms. Bartolucci enters the courtroom so meekly and sits by herself, unnoticed—but she is only in court when the prosecution is questioning witnesses. A glance towards the spot she occupied reveals an empty seat once the defense begins his interrogation. How hard this must be for her.

THE STATE CALLS: DR. LAURA BROWN

This witness appears to be a professional colleague of Jennifer Bartolucci, sister of the deceased. The defense tried to exclude her from the trial, claiming her testimony would be biased. I find her very credible.

PROSECUTOR: Please tell the jury your credentials.

DR. BROWN: I am a pain management physician. I completed my fellowship in 2002, as an interventional pain management doctor. I try to find the cause of the pain. I completed my residency in anesthesia and a fellowship in pain. I have publications on clinical research.

Q. Are you familiar with Jennifer Bartolucci?

A. She held a position with the Florida Medical Association.

Q. Did you develop a friendship?

A. No.

Q. Are you familiar with Joseph Bartolucci?

A. Yes.

Q. Did you ever meet him?

A. No. Jennifer called me.

DEFENSE: Objection.

PROSECUTOR: Please describe the nature of the call, not what she said. Did you receive a letter from the Office of the State Attorney?

DR. BROWN: Yes. I received the medical records of Joseph Bartolucci.

Q. Were you asked to do anything with the records?

A. Surrender an opinion.

Q. Are you familiar with this type of document?

A. Yes. They are lacking physician's signatures.

Q. On each, or just some?

A. On all that have a signature line. They appear to be an informed consent, like most pain management clinics. Although I've never before seen a non-overdose consent form.

DEFENSE: Objection.

The attorneys approach the bench.

PROSECUTOR: One form is called a non-overdose consent?

DR. BROWN: Yes. That I've never seen.

Q. The patient was treated with opiates, previously.

A. Good, because they are effective, but they also can cause potential risks—stop breathing.

Q. Is there a physician responsibility?

A. Yes. There must be a very important, justifiable reason for prescribing. It is also important to prescribe the smallest dose. High doses can be very dangerous.

Q. Is there an addictive nature?

A. Yes, a very strong one. Opioids are extremely addictive. Heroin is an opioid, too. Benzodiazepines can also be addictive.

Q. When a physician reviews an intake form, are there certain things doctors should be looking for?

A. Mr. Bartolucci indicated a number of different medications taken: hydrocodone, Percocet, Roxicodone, OxyContin, Methadone, MS Contin, and benzodiazepines. He had taken OxyContin up to 80 mg a day.

Q. With that information on the initial form, should that be a signal to a doctor?

A. With all of these medications, I would be led to believe that if the patient is still in pain, then the patient is not responding to this treatment. Not all pain is responsive to the opiate, and these doses were high. There is some pain that just doesn't respond. Nerve pain is poorly responsive to opioid medications.

Q. Was there an MRI?

A. It showed narrowing of L-4 L-5. This is consistent with nerve pain—sciatica (layman's term). High doses of opiates would not have been my choice. I would move on to something other than an opiate. A seizure medication lowers the threshold of an impulse.

Q. Are narcotics the only solution to control pain?

A. No. You can conduct a risk benefit analysis. Better treatment. A young person is at a higher risk for addiction. The brain is still developing into the mid-twenties. Even exposure without a genetic predisposition is a high risk. Then if you add preexisting depression.

Q. Was there any other condition for caution?

A. He had been seen by other physicians—red flag. When you see treatment by several physicians, by pain providers—in my practice we would require the records from the other physicians.

Q. Previous prescriptions. Do you see any of those records?

A. No.

Q. Here is the pharmacy record from November 24, 2008, written by Dr. W.: Percocet, sixty tablets, two per day. Percocet consists of 5 mg oxycodone and 325 mg of acetaminophen. Two per day is equivalent to 10 mg per day of oxycodone. First visit to Dr. Klein, December 10, 2008. Pain symptoms: constant, achy, penetrating sharp lower back radiating pain. Level six out of ten. Tingling, numbing, anxiety.

A. Common presentation. Doses by the other doctors were adequate. If they were not working, then other modalities should have been considered. Physical therapy, acupuncture, epidural. A treatment plan should be discussed with the patient.

Q. What was the treatment that Dr. Klein used?

A. He prescribed 150 15 mg tablets of oxycodone. This is equivalent to 75 mg per day of oxycodone. 150 for thirty days is five per day; dosage 15 mg is 15 mg times five, which equals 75 mg per day of oxycodone.

Q. Explain the problem when going from 10 mg per day to 75 mg per day.

A. That is a big jump. It could have negative consequences.

Q. Any risk factor when prescribing oxycodone with another drug?

A. Xanax and oxycodone are both CNS [central nervous system] depressants. Thirty tablets of 2 mg Xanax per day were also prescribed.

Q. January 29, 2009, Dr. Klein's progress notes. Patient reports he re-injured his back when he took a step. He has not seen Dr. W. [orthopedic doctor]. Oxycodone 30 mg, quantity one hundred-twenty, equivalent to 120 mg per day, prescribed along with Xanax 2 mg, fifteen, equivalent 1 mg per day. February 27, 2009, office visit with Dr. Klein. Pain scale five, prescribed nortriptyline, quantity thirty, 25 mg (25 mg per day) for depression and nerve pain. Dilaudid quantity 150, 8 mg. Prescription for quantity 150, 30 mg oxycodone was voided.

A. Dilaudid is much more potent than oxycodone. It is a different chemical. Dilaudid is at least four times stronger than oxycodone. When you switch from one to another, you must take into consideration how the patient will metabolize the drug. After an equal dosage is configured, then cut the dose in half before prescribing—basic pharmacy. One hundred fifty Dilaudid 8 mg is five per day; 8 mg times five equals 40 mg per day.

> Compared to oxycodone, that's quadruple the dose. It's equivalent to 160 mg per day. If 120 mg oxycodone per day was converted to Dilaudid, I would start at 20 mg per day.
>
> Q. Did you review the autopsy report?
>
> A. Yes, a few years ago. The serum drug levels were high.
>
> DEFENSE: Objection.

The judge resolves this objection, and Day Six ends.

DAY SEVEN: WEDNESDAY, SEPTEMBER 2, 2015

This morning, before the jury is brought in, the two attorneys approach the bench.

> DEFENSE: They are not calling the lab to the stand. We have no opportunity to cross-examine the cause of death. We have no way to know if a lab mistake was made. They may have done this on purpose; may be intentional.

The more the defense can get thrown out, the better it is for his case.

The jury enters. Court is in session.

THE STATE CALLS: LOUIS FISHER

Louis Fisher used to work for the DEA. Now, he has his own consulting business showing clinics how to pass a DEA inspection.

> LOUIS FISHER: I am a private consultant, with a background of thirty-one years at the DEA. I started my own business to check doctors' offices for compliance with state and federal regulations.
>
> PROSECUTOR: Are there state and federal regulations for in-house pharmacies?

DEFENSE: Objection.

LOUIS FISHER: Yes.

PROSECUTOR: Are you looking to make sure that they are in compliance?

A. I am a pharmacist by education. I rose up the ranks in the DEA and became DEA Regional Chief of Fort Lauderdale.

Q. When your business was set up, was it to make sure doctors' offices were in compliance?

A. Yes.

Q. In 2008, you visited East Coast Pain Clinic. How did that happen?

A. I was contacted by either Theo or the owner.

Q. Before wholesalers can fill orders, do they have to be in compliance? Who did you meet with?

A. I believe Theo and possibly the owner. In 2008, they were allowed to dispense drugs. The majority of what I was doing was looking at the dispensary.

Q. Did you see the dispensary?

A. Yes.

Q. In order to be in compliance, did you check records?

A. Yes. They were lacking quite a few records required by federal law. The State requires information to be displayed. I gave them some of those.

Q. Any requirements regarding printing?

A. Yes, a daily log.

Q. Were they doing that?

A. Initially, no. Then they did.

Q. Were they in compliance with receiving the medications?

A. Yes.

Q. Were they in compliance with filling prescriptions?

A. They were not. Initial script filled by tech, OK. The physician must check. This was not being done initially.

Q. When you were there, did they have a pharmacist or a pharmacy tech?

A. No.

Q. Once a physician writes a prescription should they monitor or supervise the dispensing?

A. The physician initials the bottle.

Q. Was that being done?

A. No.

PROSECUTOR: No more questions.

DEFENSE: SAME WITNESS, LOUIS FISHER

DEFENSE: We met before at the deposition.

LOUIS FISHER: Yes.

Q. Background, you worked in law enforcement.

A. Not law enforcement, DEA.

Q. So you're an investigator. No arrest power. So now you check to advise on how a clinic can get up to speed. The wholesalers wanted to hire you to inspect. They wanted to ensure the pharmacy was OK so they could sell their wares. You would tell wholesalers "don't sell to this clinic," right?

A. Yes.

I'd like to know if that ever happened.

DEFENSE: You were then hired by Jeff George. He wanted to make sure that he was running the clinic correctly. Did you do a background check on George?

LOUIS FISHER: No.

Q. You wouldn't have worked for him if you knew he had a criminal background.

A. No.

Maybe Dr. Klein should have done a criminal background check.

DEFENSE: How many clinics have you been at?

LOUIS FISHER: Dozens.

Q. Do you have an exact number?

A. No.

Q. Your job was to make sure that they were in compliance.

A. Yes.

Q. No medical check.

A. Correct.

Q. You saw that the drugs were being kept in the safe.

A. Yes.

Q. They had the Abacus system [software program]. So reports were in compliance, daily reports. Monthly inventories would be run.

A. Yes.

Q. You thought they were a typical startup clinic.

A. Yes.

Q. You noted they verified past records including MRI's. That's a good practice, right?

A. Yes.

Q. When drugs are ordered, a form goes to the wholesaler and to the DEA [222 form].

A. Yes.

Q. You said a doctor should have been checking the prescriptions. You didn't remember seeing a sign on the wall. So you don't know if there could have been a licensed pharmacist.

A. No, I didn't.

Louis Fisher was hired to inspect the business for compliance. His background as a DEA agent meant he knew what was needed to pass an inspection. He also had a pharmacist background. Theo Obermeyer and Ally Ruiz were filling the pill bottles with oxycodone and Xanax for distribution—but neither had any medical training. Louis Fisher was there to inspect the pharmacy and never checked if they had proper credentials. Interesting.

DEFENSE: You were a pharmacist, so you know about medications. If a patient develops a tolerance, medications must be increased. Can you switch to any other opiate? How would you know the conversion?

LOUIS FISHER: There are many books, charts.

Q. Do you remember the name of the wholesaler?

A. No. There were three that I worked for.

DEFENSE: No more questions.

THE STATE CALLS: DR. GERTRUDE JUSTE, ASSISTANT MEDICAL EXAMINER (ME) PALM BEACH COUNTY, FL

Dr. Juste is soft spoken and has an accent. At first, I'm afraid she will be hard to understand. But she is so thorough that I find her mesmerizing. Her tone never changes or alters, regardless of the questioning she is put through.

2ND CHAIR PROSECUTOR MICHAEL RACHEL: Dr. Juste has been a ME for Palm Beach County for seven years. How many autopsies have you performed?

DR. JUSTE: 6,000.

Q. Purpose?

A. To determine the cause of death. Prior to being a ME in Palm Beach County, I was an ME in Broward County and Washington, overall nineteen years. I attended school in Haiti, then came to the United States in 1982. I had to pass the examination in this country.

Q. How many times have you been called to testify?

A. I don't keep a log. About fifty times a year.

Q. Did you autopsy Joseph Bartolucci?

A. Yes.

Q. How do you get assigned to a case?

A. There is a schedule. Any suspicious death, any violence, anyone walks into a hospital and doesn't walk out.

Q. Do you ever go to the scene?

A. I used to. I don't anymore. We have good investigators in Palm Beach.

Q. Did you receive background information?

A. I don't think we had an investigator go to the scene, but a report was made.

Q. Identifying at-scene photos taken?

A. Yes.

Q. This is for identification—photo with toe tag.

A. Yes.

Q. Anyone else present?

A. We have assistants.

Q. What did you observe?

A. You look at the body externally, look at the eyes, look for trauma, color of body, look at mouth, teeth—nothing foreign. If no further documentation is to be made, then you open the body. When you die, the heart is no longer pumping.

Q. Can you characterize *rigor mortis*? Time of death?

A. We were told his girlfriend reported that he had been alive at a certain time. March 1, 2009, autopsy almost twenty-four hours later.

Q. Any determination to exact time of death?

A. It's always a window. We usually know when someone was last seen alive. February 28, 2009, 12:00 noon, he was alive. Some pressure point blanching was noted, so death was close to the time that he was found. Blood will pool with gravity. We estimate by pressing on the skin to see if it still blanches. If there is no blanching, the person has been dead over eighteen hours.

Q. Any facial hair, beard?

A. No. Short hair, clean.

Q. After observing the outside of the body, did you characterize the internal organs?

A. Good condition. Liver, good condition, not damaged by alcohol. Everything appeared normal.

Q. Finding of the lungs?

A. They were twice the weight as normal size. When they are heavy, they have a lot of fluid. His lungs in weight were twice the size they should have been. Cause was edema, congestion.

Q. Tissues examined?

A. No infection found. Congestion was severe.

Q. Have you ever done an autopsy on someone taking pain medications?

This is South Florida. Oh yeah.

DR. JUSTE: When someone takes these kind of narcotics, it slows down the respiratory system. Sometimes they are heard snoring. They cannot breathe—they will be heard snoring. The lungs will slow down. The heart will slow down. The lungs become heavy.

PROSECUTOR: You also take blood fluid samples. Did you send them to the lab?

A. Yes.

Q. Did you send it to the lab you always use?

A. Yes.

Q. What did you find in the GI [gastro intestinal] system?

A. Fast food contents that were undigested.

Q. Any signs of pill particles?

A. Nothing that jumped out. Sometimes you will see a partial pill. If they take a large amount, you will see them, or they will dissolve in content.

Q. You also noted the GI tract.

A. I don't normally open that unless I suspect a tumor. Stomach is always opened at the beginning of the tract.

Q. Are you familiar with OxyContin?

A. Slow motility, the bowel doesn't move as it should. People that take drugs have a problem with constipation.

Q. Results of lab report? What was the cause of death?

A. Combined drug toxicity. Hydromorphone and alprazolam. Hallmark sign, congestion of lungs. He died because he had enough drugs in his system to cause lung congestion.

Q. What was the cause of the lung congestion? What was the cause of death?

A. I called it accidental drug overdose.

PROSECUTION: No more questions.

A break for lunch was called.

DEFENSE: SAME WITNESS, DR. JUSTE

DEFENSE: We met before, at the deposition. I'm Mr. Rabin. This autopsy was March 3, 2009. Since then if your average is about fifty times a year, you've done 1,500 since then. Do you recall this specific autopsy?

DR. JUSTE: That's why we make notes, reports.

Q. As an aid to your testimony you prepare a report, correct? Things placed by the investigator, etc. You determined matter of death to be an accident?

A. Correct.

Q. You did not go to the scene? Correct? Who makes that decision? The lead detective on the scene determines whether to contact the ME office?

A. Yes and no. They will contact us, and the office will decide.

Q. Whatever Detective Sam had, he didn't require an ME on the scene.

A. Correct.

Q. Information comes to you, comes indirectly from other people. He gathers information from witnesses and conveys information. The lead investigator hears information, then he tells your investigator, then they tell you.

A. Yes and no. Our lead investigator also gathers information.

A. Refer to your notes and let me know if any information was given to Detective Sam from witnesses on the scene.

A. Looks like Jean Bartolucci.

Q. OK, my question. Did your investigator get information from Detective Sam, from witnesses on the scene? Now, some information from the scene that you would know to look for but not the detective. You didn't see the body for twenty-four hours. Things that might have been important, like is the body warm to the touch, body in air conditioning, etc. You were on call March 1, 2009. Your turn. You had a reported time of death— afternoon.

The defense attorney tells the witnesses what he thinks. He doesn't really ask them questions.

DR. JUSTE: As I said, time of death is always a window. We can determine if it is consistent with the body. Time determined when fire and rescue arrived, close of window. Time of death.

DEFENSE: Time when he was still alive, that would depend on a civilian witness. Did anyone ask you to establish a time of death?

A. Some people will tell you yes, some no.

Q. But if Detective Sam had invited you to the scene, you would be able to shrink that window.

A. I'm not sure. Maybe I could see some things—no rigor mortis, you're right. But there are so many factors. If someone died, and the temperature was lower than normal, it might delay rigor mortis. Depends on activity, temperature of environment. There are so many variables that determine less than eighteen hours or more than eighteen hours.

Q. But if a detective could reverse what a witness is saying—length of time perhaps. Is the witness truthful? But you were never asked to go down there. First thing you do is the external exam. Eyes, petechial—little tiny hemorrhages, tiny, that could be an indication of strangulation.

A. Could be, but not always.

Q. Body was somewhat stiff. Another observation in your report: *well developed, slightly obese,* and *appeared older*.

A. Yes.

Q. Why do some people appear older? Could it be alcohol? Could be activity, amount of sleep, drug use. You were given no information on drug use.

A. There were some reports regarding drug use.

Q. You were also told alcohol.

A. I didn't see that on the body.

Q. Then you cut. You indicated organs were in good condition. Look at the report. Was the liver in good condition?

I glance back to the back of the courtroom. Thank God Gina Bartolucci isn't here for this.

DR. JUSTE: Yes.

DEFENSE: Wasn't there a report of mild liver steatosis?

A. That's when fat fills liver cells. It can appear throughout the whole liver.

Q. Normally you wouldn't find that on a twenty-four-year-old.

Normally a twenty-four-year-old wouldn't be having an autopsy.

> DR. JUSTE: No, but occasionally, with an obese individual. There are other things.
>
> DEFENSE: But alcohol use can cause liver cytosis, correct?
>
> A. Yes, correct?
>
> Q. How many tubes of blood did you draw?
>
> A. Four.
>
> Q. Why do you draw?
>
> A. Various reasons.
>
> Q. You draw blood to be analyzed.
>
> A. Yes.
>
> Q. You also drew fluid from the eyes.
>
> A. Yes.
>
> Q. Did you draw urine?
>
> A. Yes. One tube.
>
> Q. Did you send the urine out?
>
> A. Yes.
>
> Q. Do you know if it was analyzed? It doesn't appear that urine was analyzed. You didn't send it out.

A. We send everything out.

Q. But it wasn't analyzed.

A. Urine is called the garbage of the body. You can find things in the urine. If you find a drug in the urine but not the blood, then they had enough time to pass the drug. The drug would not be the cause of death. Even if we find it in the urine but not in the blood, that means your body tolerated it enough to pass it through.

Q. The eye could be used to determine alcohol content. In this case you sent it out, was it analyzed?

A. No, I didn't ask them to analyze it.

Q. If someone is taking hydromorphone, alcohol potentiates it.

A. But there was no alcohol in the blood.

Q. Your blood is sent out, right? Not your lab.

A. We don't have a lab. The one we use is a forensic lab.

Q. Did you speak to them?

A. Yes.

Q. Do you know what type of analysis?

A. It is here.

Q. No, no. I'm asking you, do you know what type of machine they used?

A. No. If they find a drug they run the test three times.

Q. Were you there, doctor?

A. No.

Q. So you know how they are supposed to be done. You don't know if the machine was calibrated?

A. No.

Q. One of the questions that was raised was whether this was a suicide. From the stomach, contents travel to the small intestine. Couldn't it be possible that there could have been pills in the small intestine, but you never looked, so we wouldn't know?

A. I do know that there wouldn't be a large amount in the small intestine with none in the stomach.

As I observe all of this, I am amazed at how Dr. Juste doesn't flinch from this guy. She remains low key. Dr. Juste has science to prove her conclusion of accidental death. Establishing the possibility of a suicide might fare better for the defense attorney's client. But she knows her findings, and he isn't going to change them or cast any doubt.

DEFENSE: Hypothetical, you made a decision that it was accidental. Do you know that he lost two jobs?

DR. JUSTE: I do know that he was unemployed.

Q. He had a fight with his girlfriend. He was going to return to his mother, no car, failed rehab. He had been prescribed anti-depressants that he didn't take.

He probably would have taken them all if it was a suicide. This is just one more instance of the defense trying to exonerate the defendant, Dr. Klein, by trying to plant the seed that Joseph Bartolucci committed suicide.

DEFENSE: He was put on other serious meds, antipsychotics.

PROSECUTOR: Objection

JUDGE: Ask your question.

DEFENSE: You know there were bottles and bottles of pills at the site. From four months prior, there were pills in a pillbox, so he didn't take them as prescribed. We know he had this rough time. Were you aware of all these factors when you determined the cause of death to be accidental?

DR. JUSTE: That's not the picture I determined.

Q. But you don't know what he was thinking.

A. I do know that he took those pills for comfort.

Q. You're guessing now.

A. I don't know what was going through his mind.

Q. You were contacted by the Bartolucci family.

A. Yes.

Q. They wanted to know the status of the case. Then they contacted your boss, Dr. Bell.

A. That's possible.

Q. They wanted to know a timeline, number of pills. Did they show you a picture of the body?

A. No. Sometimes, I see pictures. Law enforcement takes them.

Q. Do you recall your deposition from March 12, 2014? That question was asked of you. Did you provide a different answer than you are answering now?

A. We didn't think I needed to view.

Q. Any reason why, to the question asked then regarding your not viewing the photo, your answer was no crime was committed? Has your answer changed?

A. No.

DEFENSE: No more questions, Your Honor.

PROSECUTOR: ON REDIRECT, DR. JUSTE

PROSECUTOR: No alcohol found in the body.

DR. JUSTE: Correct.

Q. Are you familiar with lab testing?

A. I spent six weeks working in a forensic lab as part of my training.

Q. The only drugs found in the blood were hydromorphone.

DEFENSE: Objection.

PROSECUTOR: Hydromorphone and alprazolam [Xanax]. Anything else found in the blood?

DR. JUSTE: No.

Q. Drug toxicity was found from those two drugs?

A. Yes. Fatty change in liver, little more than mild. Nothing like an orange liver that you see in alcohol abuse. I didn't see any change in the heart.

Q. Is it your opinion that blood is the best indicator of what is going on?

A. Oh, yes.

Q. Why accidental, not suicide as asked by the defense?

DEFENSE: Objection.

PROSECUTOR: How do you determine that Mr. Bartolucci was addicted to narcotics?

DR. JUSTE: You look at the medical record. Oxycodone, so he did have an addiction to narcotics. You look at the history of the person. Body was used to drugs. It happens when people go from one drug to another that you can overdose.

DEFENSE: Objection we don't need the narrative.

DR. JUSTE: Someone who has never taken hydromorphone can overdose on less.

DEFENSE: Objection. Not the question that was posed by counsel.

PROSECUTOR: Does that quantity—without giving a number. Does that level of quantity determine that it was not a suicide? Do phone calls from the family affect your opinion?

DR. JUSTE: No.

DEFENSE: Judge may we approach the bench?

JUDGE: Any other questions?

Both attorneys answer, "No, there are no more questions." The witness, Dr. Juste, is excused. A break is called. The jury leaves the courtroom.

The defense is trying to prevent someone from testifying—although I'm not able to hear who. The judge will make her decision regarding this matter at a later time.

Before the jury returns, the next witness, Christopher (Chris) Hutson, is brought into the courtroom—in shackles. As mentioned previously, the defense moved to exclude Hutson's testimony due to his proximity to Theo Obermeyer while in detention. However, the judge ruled that Hutson could testify. And now Hutson is shuffling his way across the courtroom to his seat on the witness stand, his shackles preventing him from taking normal steps. It is a bit of a reality shock. But by the time the jury sees Chris Hutson, he will be sitting down. And although mention will be made that he came here today from prison, that will not influence the jury in the same way that having seen his entrance would have.

I've learned that Chris Hutson has a twin brother named Jason. Both have known the George brothers since their youth. Chris Hutson has had other scrapes with the law, previously, and appears to me to be willing to do anything to get what he wants.

THE STATE CALLS: CHRISTOPHER HUTSON

PROSECUTOR: Where do you reside?

CHRISTOPHER HUTSON: Palm Beach County Jail, prior Jesup Georgia, federal prison.

Q. Are you serving time similar to charges, today?

A. Yes.

Q. Length?

A. Sixty months.

Q. Are you a convicted felon?

A. Yes.

Q. Any promises in return for your testimony?

A. No, ma'am.

Q. Your age?

A. Thirty-four years old.

Q. Do you know Jeff George?

A. Yes.

Q. Do you have a twin brother?

A. Yes.

Q. Did you both work for George?

A. Yes, at South Beach Rejuvenation as a sales rep. East Coast Pain. Jeff George was the owner.

Q. Do you know Theo Obermeyer, his position?

A. Manager.

Q. Somewhere around July, 2008, did you go to the clinic as a patient?

A. Yes.

Q. Did you have an injury or pain?

A. No.

Q. Did you bring anything with you?

A. Yes. An MRI.

Q. Was it your MRI?

A. No ma'am. I made a fake MRI on the Internet. I believe I said I had a motorcycle wreck. Yes, neck and back injury.

Q. When?

A. I don't know.

Q. Does it indicate on the form?

A. It says how long has it been there. I put 4-5.

Q. Just 4-5?

A. Yes.

Q. On the MRI that you indicated that you made? Where is Midtown Imaging?

A. It was in our old rejuvenation center.

Q. Did you know Dr. A?

A. No.

Q. It says he's an orthopedic. Did you alter this?

A. No ma'am. I cut and pasted it. Put my name on it.

Q. So you took this from another MRI and put your name on it? It says *MRI cervical spine*. Did you have to change anything on that?

A. No, ma'am.

Q. Everything on the MRI report was there when you took it off the Internet?

A. I didn't take it off the Internet. I believe someone that worked at Rejuvenation had them, and that's where I got that page.

Q. As you're reading through these forms, you're shaking your head.

A. To be honest with you, some of this doesn't look like my signature.

Q. Can you identify which pages were not signed by you?

A. Non-overprescribing policy, support person.

Q. Do you remember filling that out?

A. No.

Q. Do you know the name of the support person that is written there?

A. No.

Q. Any other forms that you don't think are yours? Here is another pain management agreement, a place for patient signature and physician signature. All the documents that require a physician signature, did the physician sign them?

A. No, ma'am.

Q. Once you completed the forms, you saw the doctor. What did you pay?

A. I believe it was $150.00.

Q. What date?

A. July 23, 2008.

Q. Do you have a recollection that would have been the time?

A. Yes.

Q. Did they take insurance?

A. Cash. I didn't wait in the lobby. I went with Theo and waited with him until I saw the doctor.

Q. Any special privileges?

A. Yes, ma'am. I didn't wait in line.

Q. What doctor did you see?

A. Dr. Klein.

Q. Did he ask questions about your complaint?

A. Yes.

Q. Did you change your gait?

A. On the initial exam, I was over-exaggerating. I remember he asked me to lift my leg, and I pretended not to be able to. No other doctor had me lift my leg. Dr. Klein said, "Oh, you must be one of the SE guys."

Q. Did you introduce yourself?

A. No. We were discussing my going to different doctors and what pills I was taking. I told him I was taking 240 Roxies a month, thirty Xanax.

Q. What was your interest?

A. I was going to sell them.

Q. Dr. G, she was at South Florida Pain when Chris George, Jeff George's twin brother, first opened. He asked you what Dr. G was prescribing?

A. Yes. Roxies.

Q. You were selling the Roxicodone [oxycodone]?

A. Yes.

Q. Were you asked to take a urine test?

A. I don't remember.

Q. Did you get prescriptions?

A. Yes. Roxicodone and I believe Valium.

Q. Do you remember the quantity?

A. No, I don't.

Q. Do you see this document? Do you see prescriptions that are dated on the July date?

A. Yes. July 7, 2008.

Q. Here is the document the physician Dr. Klein—210 Roxicodone, thirty Valium. Did he explain to you why he was only writing 210?

A. Yes. He said he thought 240 was too much.

Q. Do you know their policy on payment?

A. Yes. No insurance, cash or credit card only. From their other clinics, I already knew that.

Q. When you went back again, what doctor did you see?

A. Dr. Klein.

Q. Did he ask you about your level of pain? What was your best day or worst day?

A. No.

Q. Did he tell you about adverse effects?

A. No.

Q. Second visit. Date September 9, 2008. Any more forms?

A. No.

Q. Were you in the waiting room?

A. No. We had kind of an argument. He wrote for less again.

Q. Did the reason have anything to do with how you were doing? Were you doing better?

DEFENSE: Objection.

PROSECUTOR: Do you remember what he asked you?

CHRISTOPHER HUTSON: No.

Q. See where I'm pointing? *Analgesic at first visit.* Were you asked any of these questions?

A. No. I don't remember. His argument, he feels that me taking those kinds of pills there are different avenues like stretching.

Q. Did he give you any exercises?

A. No.

Q. Did you pay for the office visit?

A. Yes.

Q. Prescriptions given oxycodone 30 mg, amount 200, Valium 30. Were you taking any other drugs?

A. Yes. I was on steroids—not narcotics.

Q. When you left there that day, did you go back to East Coast Pain

Clinic? Did you have any discussion about why you skipped the month of August?

A. I don't remember.

Q. Is there any notation on the progress note?

A. I can't read it.

PROSECUTOR: No more questions, Your Honor.

The judge excuses the jury for the day. She announces that court will resume at 10:15 tomorrow morning, and a decision will be made regarding whether Dr. Goldberger (that is the name I wasn't able to hear) may testify.

DAY EIGHT: THURSDAY, SEPTEMBER 3, 2015

ATTORNEYS' DISCUSSION WITH THE JUDGE: NO JURY PRESENT

DEFENSE: Why autopsies for our testimony? The primary purpose is to analyze the cause of death. Florida court expert may not be used as a conduit to get a report in. The State chose not to call the lab in to testify. They are trying to introduce that report. The Florida Supreme Court has allowed an expert to speak about evidence not introduced—go further—only addressed in that case but not the confrontational component. This testimony would be hearsay.

PROSECUTOR: The medical examiner testimony did not attempt to get her ME report into evidence. Did not get the toxicology report into evidence. It is primarily to give them information. The end. Years later, the State got an independent lab to review the evidence. He has been deposed, and he was put on the list years ago. The case law is clear the Sixth Amendment right is not being compromised by allowing Dr. Goldberger to testify. Physicians rely on tests, MRIs, etc. We would have to go back years to change this. It is the same thing in an accident report. They rely on measurements from a crime scene. They have never been required to bring the person who took the measurements into court.

That's a good point. The defense's job is to get as much testimony thrown out as they can.

Seeking the truth? Without the jury knowing it, part of the strategy is to weaken the prosecution's case. The judge will rule on the matter later. The jury is brought in, and the trial starts for the day.

DEFENSE: RECALLS CHRISTOPHER HUTSON

DEFENSE: Yesterday, the prosecutor said you pleaded guilty in federal court. Your plea in federal court was racketeering, isn't that right? Your involvement to South East Pain Clinic was minimal. You admitted to working at an illegal anabolic steroids clinic?

CHRISTOPHER HUTSON: Yes.

Q. Weren't you in business with both George brothers? Didn't Chris George give you money to open your own MRI business?

A. I believe he gave me half.

Q. Chris George would send you patients. But that company went under. I believe there was a kickback for patient referrals. You started another business.

A. Yes.

Q. The International Marketing Finance Group. You would get a list of timeshare owners and call them. They would pay an upfront fee. Everyone was scammed. You didn't sell one timeshare. You went doctor shopping.

A. Yes.

Q. Those are the acts you admitted to. Remember the prosecutor asking you if you were ever promised anything? You said no. That's not exactly correct.

A. No, sir.

Q. The judge recommended a rehab clinic that lowered your sentence to eight years RDAP.

Residential Drug Abuse Program (RDAP) is a voluntary, 500-hour, nine- to twelve-month program of individual and group therapy for federal prisoners with substance abuse problems. It directs the Bureau of Prisons (BOP) to provide "residential substance abuse treatment (and make arrangements for appropriate aftercare) . . . for all eligible prisoners." As an incentive to get prisoners to participate, federal law allows the BOP to reduce the sentences of RDAP graduates convicted of nonviolent offenses by up to one year.

DEFENSE: Then your nine-year sentence was reduced to five years. Do you know the date?

CHRISTOPHER HUTSON: Yes. June 17, 2015.

Q. Then you come to the attention of the state. Then you had a problem because you were going back and forth, state to federal. You got a new release date, September 2, 2015. You couldn't be in RDAP. You lost your chance to get out early. At some point, you told Ms. Burns [prosecutor] this, and you asked for her help.

A. I knew she couldn't help me, and she told me that.

Q. She made phone calls for you. She told you she would write a letter. That would help you, wouldn't it?

A. Yes.

Q. You wrote a letter to the federal judge. You told him that Ms. Burns couldn't even reach the prosecutor.

A. I don't remember what I said. I was furious because I should have been out already.

Q. Here's the letter. Remember, Ms. Burns tried to contact the federal prosecutor. You went on to ask the judge, because of this back and forth and not being able to participate in the RDAP program, for a two-point reduction.

Two-point reduction: "Drugs minus two" amendment lowers all drug crimes by two offense levels.

DEFENSE: Those not eligible are serving mandatory minimum sentences, and those convicted of three strikes. That was denied, right?

CHRIS HUTSON: No. That's still in court, now.

Q. Then you asked, because I gave a deposition for the state, and I am going to trial, that you should get a reduction. And it was denied.

A. Yes.

DEFENSE: Principle 35.

Principle 35: The court may reduce a sentence if the defendant, after sentencing, provides substantial assistance in investigating or prosecuting another person.

DEFENSE: You have a brother, Jason?

CHRISTOPHER HUTSON: Yes.

Q. Your only involvement with South East Pain Clinic was to go in and lie to Dr. Klein. You brought your brother in. He's a drug addict. He doctor shops. You brought your brother in for an additional chip.

A. Yes, sir.

Q. You also paid $100,000 to Jeff George. He was going to deliver a case to you that you could give to the feds. And he scammed you.

A. Yes.

Nice friends he has.

DEFENSE: By the way. You're over there with another witness, Theo.

CHRISTOPHER HUTSON: Yes.

Q. Same unit?

A. Yes.

Q. Did anyone ever tell you not to talk about your testimony?

A. The judge yesterday said not to talk about the case.

Q. That's the first time you heard not to discuss the case?

A. I don't remember.

Q. You said that you were a doctor shopper. You would pose as a patient in pain. You filled out forms, etc. You turned to someone who was an expert.

A. Yes.

Q. The Jeff George school. He told you what to fill out on the paperwork. He told you to tell them where you had pain. He told you Dr. Klein was going to try to give you less pills. He told you how to argue with Dr. Klein.

A. Yes.

Q. Argue, beg, you're in pain. He told you Dr. Klein is straight, remember that?

A. Yes.

Q. You weren't his only pupil, right? Why don't you tell the people who else he schooled?

Many names were stated by the witness.

DEFENSE: Someone gave you a good MRI. You needed to have something to match up with what you were saying.

CHRIS HUTSON: Yes.

Q. You were armed with all this when you went to South East Pain Clinic. Jeff George would also help people get MRIs.

A. Yes.

Q. He was a full-service guy. Do you remember the date of your first visit to South East Pain?

A. No.

Q. As an employee of Jeff George, you could go to the front of the line. You weren't entitled to medication, though. You had to get those yourself. Dr. Klein's not the only person you fooled, right?

A. Right.

Q. Do you remember the first time you were interviewed?

A. Yes.

Q. You couldn't remember the name "Dr. Klein."

A. I just don't remember saying that.

Q. Did you like Dr. Klein? Was he nice?

PROSECUTOR: Objection.

CHRISTOPHER HUTSON: I don't remember.

DEFENSE: You have to remember. This was 2009; now it's 2015.

A. If you have a document, then I guess I said it, but I don't remember.

Q. You remember him doing an exam. You remember him having you touch your toes?

A. No.

Q. Do you remember raising your leg?

A. Yes.

Q. During the deposition: What do you remember about February 23, 2013? You testified under oath. Touch your toes, raised your leg, checked with rubber hammer. So you don't remember. You're not saying it didn't happen. Dr. Klein was taking notes. He's a good note taker. You asked for 240 pills. Dr. Klein said it was too much. Jeff George told you he's straight. You have to argue with him. 240 down to 210 one time, then 210 to 200. He never gave you 240, right?

A. Right.

Q. The MRI you brought to East Coast.

A. Yes.

Q. Series of consent forms.

A. Yes.

Q. Your signatures?

A. Yes.

Q. Health history, signed. Health problems, neck, back. Did you come up with that on your own or Jeff George?

A. Yes.

Q. You lied to Dr. Klein. Dr. G at South Florida Pain. You actually had gone to Dr. G?

A. Yes.

Q. Do you know if Dr. Klein ever called Dr. G?

A. I don't know.

Q. You wrote Roxies 30 mg. That was a lie. You never took them. They were to sell. You were painting a picture of pain—LIE. Did you write, in answer to the question, "Did you ever try physical therapy?" "Yes. Didn't help"? "Alternative?" "No help"? "Any other medication?" You put, "No." I guess you could have written cocaine, since you had tried that, right?

A. Yes.

Q. Have you ever been arrested? You wrote, "No." In fact, you had been arrested for trafficking cocaine. Ever arrested for a DUI? You wrote, "No."

The defense attorney proceeds through every question on the intake form. When the judge later says the trial is taking too long, and they are going to lose some of their jurors, I have to wonder, is the defense's lengthy questioning just another tactic? Strategy is very much a part of this court trial. The image of the scales of justice balancing truth and fairness is being diminished here.

DEFENSE: All to deceive Dr. Klein. "Support Person: Dean Banks."

CHRIS HUTSON: That's not my writing, not my signature.

Q. Who is Dean Banks?

A. I don't know.

Q. MRI, it says, "T-7 disk." Do you have any idea what that means?

A. No.

Q. Progress note: "Twenty-eight-year-old. Neck pain with numbness. Pain started after accident in 2004. Patient was a professional bike racer taken to Wellington Regional Hospital. Fracture left hand."

A. Yes.

Q. That did happen, right? So you weaved in some truth with the lies. Plan: "Patient on 240 oxycodone. Patient is aware that amount is too much. We will gradually reduce medications." At the time, Jeff and Chris George were in litigation. They had an argument over the main clinic. They went separate ways. How aggressive were you in arguing with Dr. Klein?

A. I might have gotten loud.

Q. He's in his seventies; you're twenty-eight. You could have knocked him down. I'm not saying you would have, but let's compare size. You're a big guy. Yet he didn't give in.

A. No. That's why I stopped going there.

DEFENSE: No more questions, Your Honor.

PROSECUTOR: ON REDIRECT, CHRISTOPHER HUTSON

PROSECUTOR: Did he really say he would wean to zero?

CHRISTOPHER HUTSON: I remember him saying that he wanted to take me off of it.

Q. Does it say here that Dr. Klein will reduce you to 180 next visit?

A. Yes.

Q. Next visit on September 18, 2008, you were given 200. Are you agreeing with counsel? Or do you really remember this conversation? First you wanted 240, and you left with 210. Now, that was thirty pills less. Did you tell him you were taking 240 for some length of time? Do you remember forms regarding the maximum amount? Read this [points to text to be read aloud]:

A. "We will be reducing slowly, no reduction more than five per month."

Q. Did he discuss he would only reduce by five per month unless you agreed?

A. No.

Q. Did he even discuss withdrawal symptoms?

A. No.

Q. Do you remember leg raising?

DEFENSE: Objection.

PROSECUTOR: Who said anything about leg lifting at the deposition? Doctor had you do leg lift. Did you say that?

CHRISTOPHER HUTSON: No.

Q. Counsel stated that when Jeff George was prepping you, he said, "Look. The guy is straight."

A. The reason I agreed to that statement was because they said "he may try to wean you down."

So the only person who said Dr. Klein was straight was his defense attorney.

PROSECUTOR: You had an appointment on July 25, then September 18. Any conversation with Dr. Klein how you got along skipping a month?

CHRIS HUTSON: No.

PROSECUTOR: No further questions, Your Honor.

A break is called by the judge. The jury leaves the courtroom. Chris Hutson, still shackled, steps out of the witness stand. The judge then announces that she has overruled the objection to the expert toxicologist testifying. A short break is taken before testimony began.

THE STATE CALLS: DR. BRUCE GOLDBERGER

Dr. Bruce Goldberger is a forensic toxicologist. He is able to confirm the finding of medical examiner Dr. Juste, who testified for the State.

PROSECUTOR: Dr. Goldberger, tell the jury a little about yourself.

DR. GOLDBERGER: I am Chief of Forensic Medicine at the University of Florida, since October 1994. My employment involves directing toxicology as well as medical examiner.

Q. Do you have hands on in the toxicology lab?

A. Yes, I did in the 1980s. Now it's a supervisory role developing a directorship for criminal toxicology: pain management, forensic toxicologist, law, medical, and legal practice.

Q. Any training in pharmacy?

A. Yes. In order to be a toxicologist, one must be trained in pharmacy, due to the action of drugs on the body. I entered the field as a student in 1982. I teach forensic toxicology and lecture on the CNS [central nervous system] drugs. How these drugs act with the brain. Medical and legal aspects. Alcohol, opioid deaths.

Q. How did you become involved in this case?

A. The State asked me to review the toxicology issues to help the State understand the reports from August, 2010.

Q. Were you provided materials to analyze?

A. The incident report, autopsy report, which included the toxicology report. I reviewed the medical report, reviewed prescription profile, and letters. The incident report provided background that led to the events.

Q. Autopsy?

A. Yes, that's the most important document, specifically the toxicology report.

Q. The prescription profile?

A. Yes.

Q. After review did you form an interpretive analysis? Explain to the jury why all are important to make an opinion. Are you familiar with the laboratory that was used?

A. Yes.

Q. Are they regularly used by the medical examiner?

A. Yes.

Q. Did you conduct an inventory of the specimens that were obtained by the ME? Blood, urine, eye fluid, gastric contents, liver? Why is a blood sample important?

A. Testing of blood is paramount.

Q. Do you have an opinion which is better, blood or urine?

A. Both are important, but blood is the most important in determining the manner of death. A comprehensive drug screen tests for alcohol, prescription drugs.

Q. Did they screen for those areas?

A. Yes. Hydromorphone and Xanax were found.

Q. Were there any indications of marijuana or cocaine?

A. No evidence.

Q. Explain pre-opiate and total opiate.

A. When hydromorphone is in the body, the body has a method of metabolizing it. So, in the end, you have a pre-drug and post- ratio. Therefore, one can tell if someone died acutely or if they were comatose for a while and then died. .069 mg/L means consumed hydromorphone before death. Second concentration can contribute to or cause death. Reckless to just look at .069 and say that's the cause of death.

Q. What did you consider for your findings?

A. My conclusion was the same as the ME. That is that Mr. Bartolucci died from ingestion of hydromorphone—total amount. He didn't die acutely. If he had died suddenly from taking a handful of pills, the numbers would be about the same. Conversely, in this case, the numbers are about half. So while he was in a drug coma, before his death his body was metabolizing the drug. There would have been an observation of lethargy, snoring while succumbing to the drug effect. Snoring is a common observation that loved ones report. Variable amounts of hydromorphone—let's say ten tabs hydromorphone found in the stomach—that would indicate suicide.

Q. You reviewed the police report.

A. Yes it was reported that half a bottle was missing. That would be a lot.

Mr. Bartolucci was given the prescription on February 27, 2009, 8 mg Dilaudid, quantity 150.

Q. If seventy-five pills were taken by Mr. Bartolucci, would those findings be the same?

A. No. The gastric level was 13.5 mg. That result is consistent with one to two tabs. If he had taken seventy-five, you would see evidence of the pills. The ME report showed no pill residue; there was food.

Q. What dose levels does Dilaudid come in? To your knowledge is that low end or high end?

A. That's high end.

Q. In your training, if someone is on one kind of drug and changes to another compound, do they always work well?

A. Both of these tablets are opiates, but everything is related to the standard of morphine. There is no way to measure how the body will tolerate. There are many charts, even apps on the phone now.

Q. Is oxycodone 30 mg the same as 8 mg hydromorphone?

A. No. Hydromorphone is about ten times the potency of morphine.

Q. So, oxycodone 30 mg quantity 150, hydromorphone 8 mg quantity 150. Are they equal?

DEFENSE: Objection.

JUDGE: Overruled.

DR. GOLDBERGER: No, they are not equal. I'm not a physician, but I teach how to use the charts. Whatever the chart says, cut that dose in half or one quarter of the dose.

PROSECUTOR: And monitoring?

A. Yes. Repeated visits to insure they are stable on these very potent opioids.

Q. When the drugs are combined, for instance, hydromorphone and Xanax?

A. Yes. It's widely known now that when mixing the opiate and benzodiazepines it increases the likelihood of overdose. It slows the breathing and some believe affect the integrity of the airway. It causes an accumulation of fluid in the trachea that sounds like snoring.

Q. Based on your review, were you able to form an opinion?

A. Yes. The combination of hydromorphone and Xanax was lethal to Mr. Bartolucci.

No wonder the defense did not want this witness to testify.

DEFENSE: SAME WITNESS, DR. GOLDBERGER

DEFENSE: We get a copy of all the cases that you have been deposed on. 600 times. Two-thirds criminal cases, one-third civil. In 400 criminal cases, that's ninety-five percent, you were a witness for the State. When you testified earlier that you kind of split as far as your findings for the State or defense, that's not actually true, is it?

DR. GOLDBERGER: As a toxicologist, we get called in by the State.

Q. You agree with the ME finding. Is that correct?

A. Yes. It was an accidental death.

Q. Nothing you have done changes that opinion. You are familiar with Xanax. You even stated to Mrs. Bartolucci and Mr. Bartolucci's sister that your dog took Xanax.

A. My dog took Valium. But my wife took Xanax.

Q. So basically a lot of people take Xanax, wouldn't you agree?

A. Yes.

The defense attorney is still trying to make a fool of any professional who does not agree with him. Unfortunately, he is right. These drugs are overused. The drug companies keep promoting the need for them, and people follow like sheep.

DEFENSE: What was the dosage?

DR. GOLDBERGER: 2 mg, take a ½ tab every night.

Q. So the dose was 1 mg. Is 1 mg a lot?

A. No.

Q. Is it excessive?

A. No. Tolerance defines how a body reacts to repeated drugs. First time sluggish; second and repeated times, less effect.

Q. The human body, if never taken before, one opiate can kill someone.

A. It can. Depends on the dosage.

Q. So a chronic patient can take two, three, four, maybe ten times the amount?

A. I'm not going to say ten times the amount.

But of course, we know why the defense attorney wants the witness to say "ten times the amount." The amount prescribed by his client, Dr. Klein, should have been cut in half. The dosage Dr. Klein ordered for Joseph Bartolucci was lethal. Deaths from opiates are not just the result of non-medical use; they are also the result of over-prescribing by doctors. But the jury hears what the defense attorney (who is not under oath) interjects, not just how the witness responds.

> DEFENSE: Part of that tolerance is that it is safe to take larger doses. In this case, this patient was not opiate naive, was he? In the medical record he went from 15 mg to 30 mg. In the record it shows he took 250 mg per day.
>
> DR. GOLDBERGER: I don't recall that.

The defense attorney brings the record for him to read.

> DR. GOLDBERGER: Yes, that is correct. In July of 2008, Roxie 250 mg per day.
>
> DEFENSE: Let's talk about the lab. You described in our deposition that it was adequate. You know it does not have the credentials that the University of Florida has. Do you know anything about the analyst that handled the tests?
>
> A. No.
>
> Q. Do you know about the chain of custody?
>
> A. Of course. Anyone who analyzes a sample or allocate, initials them.
>
> Q. But you don't know how they did a test, if their machine was calibrated.
>
> A. I accepted their finding.
>
> Q. You don't know if it was the same blood that was extracted.

The defense attorney is really reaching now.

> DR. GOLDBERGER: I think the inference was there based on what was found.
>
> DEFENSE: Let's talk about your deposition in Gainesville. You cannot

tell this jury how many pills were taken?

A. Correct.

Q. Conversion tables. 2009 the decedent died. Physicians were required to use conversion tables; in fact, they use them still today. Physicians use tools. You're suggesting that physicians ought to be a little more cautious.

A. Yes.

Q. The purpose of a conversion chart is so that if you are on an opiate, you don't just come off it.

A. Well you do in treatment; it's not lethal. It's uncomfortable. If on an opioid, and it's no longer available, it hurts. Withdrawal from benzodiazepines, on the other hand, can be lethal.

Q. You never met Mr. Bartolucci?

A. No.

Q. You don't know what his tolerance was?

A. No.

Of course, he does have a death certificate.

> DEFENSE: The prosecution asked you about suicide. You want to know what's going on in an individual's life.
>
> DR. GOLDBERGER: Yes, there are many questions.
>
> Q. Yes, all of those factors must be considered before rendering an opinion. Committed suicide or didn't.
>
> A. Yes. Or didn't.

Q. You testified that hydromorphone was the cause of death based on everything. Mr. Bartolucci is dead. No other cause of death. No aneurysm. So the most obvious answer, what was found in the blood. Again you don't know how many pills he took.

A. Correct.

DEFENSE: No further questions.

PROSECUTOR: ON REDIRECT, DR. GOLDBERGER

PROSECUTOR: Any questions on cross that caused you to change your opinion?

DR. GOLDBERGER: No.

Q. Hydromorphone, one tablet every four hours. So could be six a day?

A. Yes.

Q. If someone filled a prescription at 4:00 p.m. and is still awake at midnight, they could have taken two pills?

A. Yes.

Q. You were asked about suicide?

A. Yes. There were a number of psychosocial issues. But I didn't see any evidence of suicide.

Q. Regarding the work you've done on opioid deaths, if someone is trying to commit suicide, would they take the time to cut a pill in half?

A. No.

PROSECUTOR: No more questions, Your Honor.

DAY NINE: FRIDAY, SEPTEMBER 4, 2015

No traffic today. It's Labor Day weekend, and I make the trip in one hour. Dr. Klein went through the metal detectors downstairs right ahead of me. We could have ridden in the same elevator, but I chose not to. He was by himself.

THE STATE CALLS: ALEJANDRO PINO

Alejandro Pino is dressed in long khaki shorts. He is a little bit overweight, all smiles. I will learn during his testimony that he once was a drug seeker, but is now clean. The opiate is an addiction that is very hard to overcome. There are many relapses. I hope and pray he stays clean. He is a very likable young man.

PROSECUTOR: What do you do for a living?

PINO: I manage a halfway house.

Q. Do you counsel?

A. Yes, mostly for drug abuse. Prior to that, I worked in a restaurant.

Q. Are you a recovering addict?

A. Yes.

Q. Have you met Jeff George?

A. No.

Q. Are you familiar with Dr. Klein?

A. Yes.

Q. Are you familiar with East Coast Pain Clinic?

A. Yes, ma'am.

Q. Do you remember when you visited the clinic?

A. 2008, 2009.

Q. Did you fill out forms?

A. I believe so.

Q. Here are the intake forms dated January 29, 2009. Your name? Your handwriting?

A. Yes.

Q. What was your purpose?

A. I was in active addiction.

Q. Were you seeing other doctors at the time?

A. No.

Q. What drugs were you seeking?

A. Roxy, Xanax.

Q. Do you remember when you first started pills?

A. Yes. After a car accident in 2004. I got addicted.

Q. How did you know how to go to East Coast Pain Clinic?

DEFENSE: Objection!

PROSECUTOR: Did you hear about them on the news or in the paper?

ALEJANDRO PINO: No.

Q. When you went there, did you bring something with you?

A. Yes. I took an MRI.

Q. Was there a charge for the office visit? How much?

A. I don't recall.

Q. Do you know if they took insurance from you?

A. No, I paid cash.

Q. What were you prescribed in 2004 after the car accident?

A. Xanax, Roxies.

Q. Were you being truthful when you answered the questions on the forms?

A. I don't remember. I was just drug seeking and answering the questions.

Q. The MRI that you took, was that your MRI?

A. Yes.

Q. Was that ordered by a different doctor?

A. I believe so.

Q. Have you ever had physical therapy, and did it help? You answered, Yes, to both questions. Was that true? Had you had those treatments?

A. No.

Q. Had you been to Good Samaritan and St. Mary's hospital? You signed a consent for records.

A. I believe so.

Q. Did you meet with a doctor and have a conversation?

A. Yes. Dr. Klein.

Q. Did you go there more than once?

A. I can't recall.

Q. Were you under the influence when you went?

A. Absolutely.

Q. Additional notes: Thirty-two-year-old chef for Donald Trump. Is that where you worked?

A. Yes.

Q. What drugs were you hoping to get?

A. Xanax and Roxies.

Q. Do you remember having a discussion that the amounts of your drugs were too high?

A. I don't remember.

Q. Would that have been something that you would have wanted to hear?

A. No.

Q. You took with you a copy of a prescription prescribed by Dr. C. You also told him Xanax, oxycodone 30 mg amount 240. Did you receive prescriptions from Dr. Klein?

These are copies of prescriptions that you received: Dr. Gerald Klein 1/29/09 oxycodone 30 mg 240, Xanax 2mg 90; 2/26/09 oxycodone 30 mg, 230 Xanax 2 mg 90; 03/26/09 Xanax 2 mg 90, oxycodone 30 mg 230. Were you still drug-seeking in March?

A. Yes.

Q. Were you ever court ordered to go to CARP [Comprehensive Alcoholism Rehabilitation Program], an agency located in Palm Beach County, Florida, for alcohol and drug abuse?

A. Yes.

Q. Did Dr. Klein have a conversation that he was going to wean you?

A. I don't remember.

Q. Would you have gone back if he told you he was going to wean you?

A. No.

Q. Did you ever receive a referral to a rehab center from Dr. Klein?

A. No.

Q. Do you remember going to St. Mary's Hospital?

A. No.

Mr. Pino is shown a fax from St. Mary's Hospital. It says, *Patient is detoxing from Roxy, Xanax and cocaine; also seen at Good Samaritan Hospital. Tremors.*

PROSECUTOR: Do you see the fax sent from St. Mary's to East Coast?

ALEJANDRO PINO: Yes. February 12, 2009.

Q. When you went to your appointment on February 26, 2009, did Dr. Klein ever discuss St. Mary's hospital with you? When you went there after going to detox?

A. No.

Q. Did Dr. Klein or anyone else discharge you from East Coast?

A. No.

Q. Did you decide to quit going?

A. Yes.

Q. Back to the March 26, 2009, appointment [looks at progress notes]: Patient went to CARP for detox? And you still left March 26, 2009 with prescriptions for oxycodone and Xanax?

A. Yes.

Prosecution: No more questions.

DEFENSE: SAME WITNESS, ALEJANDRO PINO

DEFENSE: You and I met at the deposition—one time. How many times have you met with the prosecutor? You would agree you have poor recollection of the time you were at East Coast Pain?

ALEJANDRO PINO: Yes.

Q. You have no recollection, in fact. I don't even think you recognize Dr. Klein.

A. He's in the middle, over there [points].

Q. But you kind of know that's who he is. Your MRI showed information from a car accident. Additionally, you have been given immunity from the State?

A. Yes.

Q. Mr. Frazier told you that you were an important witness in this case.

A. Yes.

Q. Mr. Frazier told you that you went to CARP, and that Dr. Klein never even talked to you about that.

A. I don't remember.

Q. What's your understanding about why you're here today?

A. My understanding, I guess, is that they say I'm a prime witness against Dr. Klein.

Q. It's clear that you have memory issues. In the deposition, you said you don't even know Dr. Klein. One thing you wouldn't admit to is that you were the best liar you could be to get those pills. And you lied to Dr. C., too. You used the car accident to your advantage.

A. Yes.

Q. Now, the MRI, this is the truth, this is yours. Mild-moderate disc bulging L5, L1-L2, L2-L3, L4-L5, most severe L1-L2. The pharmacy record shows that Dr. C. gave you an additional opiate that Dr. Klein didn't give you. In summary you had been to two or three other doctors. You knew what to say. You were, in your own words, the best liar in order to get your drugs. Do you know there is a law requiring patients to be honest with their doctor?

A. I don't know.

Q. You really were in pain. You needed those drugs, right?

A. Yes.

Q. You are on a good path, now.

A. Yes.

Q. Dr. Klein didn't help you on either path, right? You were drug seeking of your own free will.

A. Yes.

Q. The prosecutor asked you all kinds of questions. Were you examined? When in fact if someone had told you there was a blue monkey in the room you wouldn't have known!

A. Correct.

Q. Note from January 29, 2009, says low back pain. Is that where you were injured?

A. Yes.

Q. Five years' duration, accident, thrown from car. Do you know if you were thrown from the car?

A. I don't remember.

Q. Next line: St Mary's trauma four weeks. This is information that would have had to have come from you, right? Patient lost feeling back of leg, back of arm.

A. I don't remember.

Q. I'm reading from Physician Impression: Low back pain, multiple levels of bulging discs, so this could have come from you or Dr. Klein. Plan to discontinue OxyContin 80 mg. You were getting thirty 80 mg tabs. Replace oxycodone 240 30 mg and Xanax. Patient told of plan to decrease at next visit.

Next note, February 26, 2009: Patient off OxyContin 80 mg two times per day. Patient said he felt the effect at beginning of the month. You wouldn't remember but it's written here.

The attorney for the defense is sarcastic and intimidating. This particular patient came about his addiction honestly. It is the opiate that is so highly addictive leading to this path; not all addicts started out on the joy ride.

DEFENSE: Patient taking oxycodone ten times a day. Patient seen at Good Samaritan Hospital in 2004. So, if records had come in, Dr. Klein must not have seen. You would not have known when the record was put in your file. Third note, March 03, 2009: Patient went to CARP for detox. Then, next to it, patient was court ordered. Why did you go to court?

ALEJANDRO PINO: I wanted to get off of drugs.

DEFENSE: No. The real reason was because you wanted to have visitation with your kids. You went to CARP, got what you wanted—partial custody. You told Dr. Klein you wanted custody of your child. He wrote, "Appears honest." You obviously discussed it with Dr. Klein. He wouldn't have known that. Now, let's look at the notes.

DEFENSE (READING FROM THE PATIENT'S FILE: PLAN OF CARE): Same Oxycodone this month. Plan to reduce next month. He told you he was going to decrease you and you never went back. Do you remember pages 19-20 of the deposition? The investigator told you because you seemed like somebody who was sincere and wanted to get off drugs, but Dr. Klein didn't discuss it with you. We now know that's not true. Six years clean, February 7, 2010. You made that decision. If you had wanted to get drugs, you would have gotten them. If we locked up every doctor in the country, you would have gotten drugs.

PROSECUTOR: Objection.

The truth is, until recently, every pain pill was put there by a physician. This is a physician-prescribed epidemic. Whether pills end up in someone's hand from a medicine cabinet, or they got them from a friend, pain pills originate from a physician. This has been allowed to happen due to lax laws and the BOM allowing high-prescribing doctors to maintain their licenses. I once had a mother share with me that after her seventeen-year-old daughter took just one quarter of a pain pill offered to her by her friend after she broke up with her boyfriend, the young girl began frequenting pill mills. She told staff members that she hurt herself falling off a horse—or whatever story was needed to ensure she left with pills. However, she could *not* have gone into Publix and bought a beer. At the grocery story, they check ID. Yet no such requirement was in place in the pill mills. So yes, they lied. But it didn't matter as long as they had the money.

DEFENSE: You never went in appearing like you were intoxicated. You knew how to hide that. Back to March 26, 2009, note, left off one line. "Got custody of child" appears sincere. Next line: We will keep close scrutiny with patient as a result of this conversation or whatever else happening in your life. You never went back.

ALEJANDRO PINO: Yes.

Q. During the time you were seeking drugs, you were able to function, cook for Mr. Trump.

A. Yes.

Q. Same as you would be able to appear before a doctor as if you were not under the influence.

A. Yes.

DEFENSE: No more questions.

PROSECUTOR: ON REDIRECT, ALEJANDRO PINO

PROSECUTOR: Lack of memory; was it true that when you met with the investigators the time was close to the event? Did you tell the truth?

ALEJANDRO PINO: Yes.

Q. Regarding your memory of Dr. Klein having a discussion with you. Would it help if you looked at the statement from 2011? Here is the deposition between you and Investigator Frazier (read line seven, to yourself). Do you remember that now? Did you say, in 2011, to the investigator that Dr. Klein was cutting back your medications? "They are cracking down." Who would that be? The DEA? So he told you because the DEA . . .

DEFENSE: Objection.

PROSECUTOR: Was it more for your health, or because of the DEA?

ALEJANDRO PINO: It was just regulations that he could not give me that amount.

Q. Since you were off OxyContin 80 mg, you were taking oxycodone eight to ten per day.

A. Don't remember.

Q. Do you see any notes of that discussion? Do you see anything remotely like counseling or of taking your drugs as prescribed? Did he ask you how did you get through the month if you were taking eight to ten pills a day?

DEFENSE: Objection.

PROSECUTOR: Do you see anything noted to address that?

ALEJANDRO PINO: No.

Q. Do you have any recollection? Or is it noted that he wanted to see you before once a month?

A. No.

Q. Any notation as to giving you for a partial month and then bringing you back?

DEFENSE: Objection.

PROSECUTOR: Did you leave with a full prescription?

ALEJANDRO PINO: Yes.

PROSECUTOR: No more questions.

There are many tragic incidents—including death—involving children being cared for by parents who are under the influence of drugs. The DCF (Department of Children and Family Services) is overwhelmed. They cannot handle the load. The prosecutor did not bring this up. The witness, Alejandro Pino, had discussed with the doctor that he went to CARP to gain custody of his child, and that he was taking eight to ten oxycodone a day, along with Xanax. Yet he still left the clinic that day with prescriptions.

THE STATE CALLS: JASON HUTSON

The last witness called is Jason Hutson. He is the twin brother of Chris Hutson, who testified earlier in this trial. When the prosecutor calls Jason Hutson, though, he isn't there. Judge Karen Miller calls a short recess but is not happy with the prosecutor. She gives prosecutor Barbara Burns a lashing for not having her next witness ready. These benches get hard, so I walk out of the courtroom—but I hear the prosecutor and her assistant get word that Jason Hutson is downstairs going through security. (When I speak with her, Barbara Burns tells me it always takes Jason Hutson a long time to get through security because he has to carry so many medications with him.)

He is very flustered and nervous by the time he reaches the courtroom. He is extremely thin, looks to be less than 100 pounds. (Compared to his muscular, robust brother, Chris, Jason looks like a fragile bird.) But he is here. The prosecutor tells him to calm down, take a few breaths; it is OK. This after she has been berated by the judge for Jason Hutson's delay—but you would never know that had occurred, judging by her calm demeanor with her witness.

Assistant State Attorney Burns begins by asking Jason Huston to introduce himself to the jury. He states his name. She asks where he has worked in the past. He says he was a bartender and worked for his brother. He worked at the steroid business.

PROSECUTOR: Do you remember when?

JASON HUTSON: Maybe 2007.

Q. Are you a recovering addict?

A. Yes. Almost four years.

Q. What drugs do you currently take?

A. Dilantin [anti-seizure], Klonopin [anti-seizure], and Subutex.

Subutex, a brand of buprenorphine, taken as prescribed, is an important part of pharmacological treatment for heroin or opiate addiction.

PROSECUTOR: Prior to 2012, what were you taking?

JASON HUTSON: Oxycodone [opiate], Xanax [anti-anxiety].

Q. What dosages?

A. Three to four pills a day.

Q. What was the dosage of the drug?

A. Roxicodone 30 mg.

Q. Was the amount you were taking enough to put you under the influence?

A. Yes.

Q. How long were you taking the drugs?

A. Eight years.

Q. How do you know Jeffrey George?

A. Through my brother.

Q. Do you know Theo Obermeyer?

A. Yes, we went to high school together.

Q. Did you work for Jeffrey George?

A. I carried files.

Q. How do you know Dr. Klein?

A. Because I went to East Coast Pain Clinic.

Q. Do you know who owned East Coast Pain Clinic?

A. Yes.

Q. Do you know when you went?

A. Are you inquiring about the date and month?

Q. I'll show you paperwork to refresh your memory [shows paperwork]. Do you recognize this paperwork?

A. Yes.

Q. Can you read me the date?

A. August 01, 2008.

Q. Did you take anything with you?

A. Oh, an MRI.

Q. The MRI you took with you, was it real?

A. No. I paid Jeff George $500 for the MRI.

Q. Do you know if your brother went to East Coast Pain Clinic as a patient?

A. Yes.

Q. Anyone else?

A. Yes, my mother.

Q. Did you go by yourself?

A. I went with my mother.

Q. Did you meet with Dr. Klein?

A. Yes.

Q. Did you both meet with Dr. Klein at the same time, in the same room?

A. Yes, ma'am.

Q. Do you remember what you paid?

A. Yes. $75.00.

Q. Did your mother pay, too?

A. Yes.

Q. How did you pay?

A. Cash.

Q. Do they take insurance?

A. No.

Q. Did Dr. Klein do a physical exam on you or your mother?

A. No.

Q. Did you let Dr. Klein know what you wanted?

A. Yes.

Q. Did Dr. Klein know who you were?

DEFENSE: Objection.

PROSECUTOR: Did the doctor know who you were?

JASON HUTSON: He knew my last name. He knew who I was.

Q. Did he ask if your mother was Chris Hutson's mother?

A. Yes.

Q. Did you get a benefit for working for Chris George?

A. Yes. I only paid $75 for a visit.

Q. After being in the room with the doctor for a few minutes, did you get a prescription?

A. Yes. Roxie 30 mg, quantity 240; Xanax 2 mg.

Jason Hutson seems to be guessing. The prosecutor shows Exhibit 8, paperwork.

PROSECUTOR: Roxicodone 30 mg 240 is circled. Why?

JASON HUTSON: Cause that's what I wanted.

Witness is shown a copy of the prescriptions received that day. The prescriptions are oxycodone 30 mg, quantity 210 and Xanax 2 mg, quantity 90.

PROSECUTOR: Look at this for me. Is this the MRI report? The one you paid $500 for?

JASON HUTSON: Yes.

Q. What did you do to make it look like yours?

A. Copied and pasted my name on the top.

Q. Do you know who Dr. W. is, whose name is the ordering physician for the record?

A. No.

Q. Did you sign a consent form so they could order the medical records?

A. Yes.

Q. On the initial paperwork, where it says health problems, did you put none?

A. Yes, ma'am.

Q. Did you put "five car accidents"?

A. Yes.

Q. There is a question: "Have you ever been to rehab?" You circled, No.

A. Correct.

Q. There is a question further down on this form that asks, "At what age did you enter rehab?" Your answer is twenty-one. Did you go back again?

A. Yes, ma'am.

Q. Did you go alone or was someone with you?

A. My mother was with me.

Q. Did you go into the exam room at the same time?

A. Yes.

Q. Was a physical exam done on you with your mother there, or on your mother with you there?

A. No.

Q. Prescriptions Xanax 2 mg, oxycodone 30 mg, quantity 210. Next appointment, October 01, 2008. When you and your mother visited the clinic, did the doctor come in each time?

A. Yes, ma'am.

Q. Prescriptions for that day: Xanax 2 mg, quantity 30; oxycodone 30 mg, quantity 200. Did the doctor ever counsel you on weaning medication?

A. No, ma'am.

Q. Can you read this, labeled, "Physicians Note," same page for the August 28, 2008, visit but at the bottom of the page. Date October 1, 2007 [sic, year incorrect]. Is this your handwriting?

A. No, ma'am.

Q. We have received records from Wellington Regional Hospital. Did you ever see a Dr. R?

A. No, ma'am.

Witness appears confused.

PROSECUTOR: "Patient was told to wear a back brace." Were you ever told to wear a back brace?

JASON HUTSON: No, ma'am.

Q. "Patient has custody of daughter's three children." Were you old enough to have a daughter who had three children?

A. No, ma'am.

Q. Did Dr. Klein do a physical examination on August 28, 2008, or October 1, 2008?

A. No, ma'am.

Q. Did he check your range of motion? Your gait? Anything like that?

DEFENSE: Objection, Your Honor. Counsel has already established that no physical exam was done.

PROSECUTOR: No more questions.

The defense attorney has just stated on record that no physical exam was done. Nice admission on his part. His client, Dr. Klein, did no exam on either patient. The defense attorney has work to do.

DEFENSE: SAME WITNESS, JASON HUTSON

DEFENSE: Mr. Hutson, we met one time when I took your deposition. How many times did you meet with the prosecutor?

JASON HUTSON: About three times.

Q. You also met with the DEA because of your brother, Chris. They asked you to help them for your brother, Chris?

A. Yes.

Q. You were going to make cases to get your brother's sentence reduced.

A. Yes, sir.

Q. You were also offered money, were you not?

A. Yes.

Q. You were upset because your brother's sentence was not reduced. You were angry, and you didn't even get paid. Is that correct?

A. Yes, sir.

Q. You are here today to try to get your brother's sentence reduced. Is that correct?

A. Yes.

Q. You were told you wouldn't get prosecuted for doctor shopping, right?

A. Yes.

Q. Now let's talk about the forms you filled out. Five car accidents, that in fact is true, isn't it?

A. Yes.

Q. Now, let's talk about the medications that you're currently on that you mentioned. Dilantin 100 mg for seizures, Klonopin for anxiety, sleep.

A. No, that's anti-seizure.

Q. OK. And I believe there were two more?

A. No. One.

Q. What is the other one? I thought you said four all together.

A. The other one is Subutex.

Q. Subutex. OK. You do have other issues. Your sister had died. By the way did she have three children?

A. She has four.

Q. Now, five car accidents, serious, they required hospitalizations. Did you get 180 stitches in your head?

A. No.

Q. You didn't go to the hospital and get 180 stitches?

A. Yes.

Q. Deposition page 38: "Pouring rain; yield, guy behind me ran into me, injuries L4 L5, bad whiplash, shoulder."

A. I didn't get the L4 L5 from that accident.

Q. Oh. So you confused accidents?

A. Yes.

Q. You had major pain from that accident.

A. Minimal.

Q. You said you cracked your shoulder.

A. I don't remember.

Q. You swore under oath. You were sworn in.

A. I don't remember.

Q. Just like today, you were sworn in and promised to tell the truth.

The defense attorney starts flipping through the pages of the deposition and appears to be highly annoyed.

JASON HUTSON: You're confusing me.

DEFENSE: You said in the deposition that you were taking medication.

A. No, sir.

Q. Well. Again, you either lied then, or you're lying now.

Defense Attorney Rabin hands the deposition to the witness and tells him to start reading from pages 2006-2008.

JASON HUTSON: The page is blank.

DEFENSE [screaming]: Well then go to 2007, wherever you need to read to refresh your memory.

I don't know if Attorney Rabin is deliberately trying to fluster the witness with his own mistake about page numbers. But I am glad the prosecutor corrects him.

PROSECUTOR: Do you mean pages 207 and 208?

DEFENSE: OK. I mean 207, 208. OK. So does that refresh your memory? You were, in fact, using drugs the day of your deposition.

The defense attorney appears furious at the witness. He makes no apology for the confusion he caused.

JASON HUTSON: Subutex...

DEFENSE: That is a drug, is it not? In fact, that is an opiate.

A. It is an opiate blocker.

Q. You described using Subutex and being a lot less high then you were when you gave your deposition in 2011.

A. Yes, sir. That's where I was getting confused.

Q. You said your shoulder was split. Was it or not?

A. No.

Q. Why did you lie about having surgery?

A. Because it was dislocated. It wasn't surgery.

Q. Deposition February 18, 2014: "After two months in a sling, I had surgery." OK, you see this book? You see it says State of Florida versus ... Before you start giving answer.

A. I don't remember being placed under oath.

Q. No. Do you think this deposition just fell out of the sky?

The defense attorney continues badgering the witness. He is loud and intimidating.

DEFENSE: So far you said you didn't have surgery, but in a deposition you said you did. You were in that sling for eight months?

JASON HUTSON: I was in a sling for eight months?

Jason Hutson seems confused.

DEFENSE: Back when you gave this deposition, you said cracked shoulder. You said you were in a sling for eight months. Do you know you could be arrested for lying under oath? Second accident: Palm Beach Lakes. "Guy ran a red light. We t-boned." You were injured.

JASON HUTSON: Mild.

Q. You had legitimate pain.

A. Yes.

Q. Why would you say mildly? Now, third accident when was that?

A. I don't remember the exact date or month.

Q. Well you had a third accident in Broward County. "Guy ran a red light." Fourth accident, you were side swiped.

A. I had no injury.

Q. Were you still suffering pain from the earlier accident? In 2010, on Griffin Road, you were rear-ended. Is that when you got 180 staples in your head?

A. You're confusing me.

Q [screaming]. Griffin Road, turnpike, rear-ended. Is that when you got staples?

A. That's when I had seizures.

Q. You got staples from an accident, not from seizures. You and I didn't meet three times so I could go over the questions with you like the prosecutor.

A. You're confusing me. I have epilepsy. You're confusing me. Can you lower your voice and be calm?

The defense attorney begins mocking the witness, speaking in a voice that is much, much lower—barely above a whisper. This is brutal to watch. I feel like I am being sucked into a cyclone that I will never get out of. Even just as an observer in the murder trial today, I feel traumatized. I can't imagine how Jason Hutson must be feeling.

> DEFENSE (whispering): OK. I am asking you these questions for the first time. OK. The accident where you injured your shoulder, split your leg. Bulging L4 L5 causing you pain—major. In the first accident, with the dislocated shoulder or injured, whichever you're going with today, the accident caused you major injury, did it not?
>
> JASON HUTSON: Yes, sir.
>
> Q. You had five accidents. In fact, you could have used your own MRI. You even said that. Do you remember that?
>
> A. No, sir.

Defense starts flipping through the book again, clearly annoyed.

> DEFENSE: Page 181 line 20, talking about your MRI. You're saying if you had your own MRI, how much it would justify you to get the drugs you were seeking? Your answer: "120 Roxies and some Xanax."
>
> JASON HUTSON: I don't recall.
>
> Q. Well it doesn't matter if you remember it or not. You said it in your deposition.
>
> JUDGE: Take baby steps.
>
> DEFENSE: I'm trying, Your Honor.

What the defense is *trying* to do is crush the witness.

> DEFENSE: What were you talking about when you said, "just wanted to feel good, just wanted pain to go away"?

JASON HUTSON: I don't remember.

Q. You said it. It's here. You have other health issues. Mental health issues.

A. No.

Q. You were treated by Dr. R in 2001. Bipolar, schizophrenia. Five times. When was the first time you were treated for mental illness? PTSD, bipolar, schizophrenia? Do you remember?

A. Not the schizophrenia.

Q. Now are you saying that you weren't diagnosed with schizophrenia?

A. Not that I recall. [Witness's voice is low, almost inaudible.]

Q. Did you give me an answer?

A. Yes, sir.

Q. On East Coast clinic form: Question: "Have you ever been treated for mental illness?" You lied?

A. Yes.

Q. As a matter of fact, you even lied when the state attorney asked you if you've ever been diagnosed with mental illness.

Witness starts to say something about Broward County. The judge asks him to stop talking, please, and calls the attorneys to the bench. Then the defense begins questioning the witness again, his demeanor improved.

DEFENSE: I want to straighten out, if I can, the different times you've been interviewed. The first time, you went with your brother, Chris. Date, March 4, 2011. This is called a report.

JASON HUTSON: May I see it?

Q. Not right now. They were cops.

The defense wants to let Jason Hutson know that he, the defense attorney, is still the one in charge.

JASON HUTSON: I don't remember talking to cops.

DEFENSE: You don't know that the DEA are cops? They asked you questions. You answered. That's a report. The second time you met with the prosecutor, the one you called "Barbara," earlier.

A. I'm sorry. I apologize for that.

Q. No, I'm sorry. Call her whatever you want. That's called a statement. The third time was with Investigator Frazier, with a woman typing. That's a deposition. So this is how I will refer to them from now on.

A. Thank you very much.

Q. Now, at the deposition, you lied to them when you were asked about mental health. By the way, you know that's a crime, right? Lying to a federal agent is a crime. Why did you lie?

A. I didn't lie. I was confused.

Q. Investigator Frazier asked the question, "Have you ever been diagnosed with schizophrenia?" Your answer was, "No." "Bipolar?" Answer, "No." "Any mental illness?" The witness that was in the deposition, which was you, answered, "Dr. Rodriguez diagnosed in 2001."

A. That was fourteen years ago, and I was on drugs.

Q. It says Dr. Rodriguez, in 2001, diagnosed you with PTSD, Bipolar. You answered this, and schizophrenia. Would you like to see it? [Shows Jason Hutson the document.]

A. Yes. OK, sir.

Q. You see I didn't make it up right?

A. Yes.

Q. So, we can now say that Dr. Rodriguez diagnosed you in 2001. He diagnosed you with PTSD, bipolar, and schizophrenia?

A. Yes, sir.

Q. When did you start using drugs?

A. 2001.

Q. Would it be fair to say that your taking drugs interferes with your ability to think?

A. And my sister dying, my dad dying, my uncle dying in New York. He was hit by a taxicab.

Q. In 2001, do you remember where you were living and what drugs you were taking?

The defense attorney has gone back to his loud, high pitched, intimidating tone.

JASON HUTSON: No.

The attorney continues to ask the same questions, unrelentingly. He is screaming.

DEFENSE: In 2002, do you remember where you were living and what drugs you were taking?

JASON HUTSON: No.

This continues for 2003, 2004, 2005, 2006, 2007. The witness's voice is getting lower and lower, and he is turning his head to the side and sobbing. The judge calls for a short break.

After the jury leaves the room, the judge asks the witness if he needs her to call 911 or the paramedics. He says, "No, I just need to calm down." After a short break, with the jury still out of the room, the judge asks the attorneys what they would like to do about this witness. By agreement of counsels, Jason Hutson is going to be stricken as a witness.

The defense also makes sure the State's expert witness, Dr. Rubenstein, won't mention the name Jason Hutson. The State acknowledges agreement. Defense also requests that the witness be called back into the courtroom so he, the defense attorney, can state in front of the jury that he did not mean to embarrass the witness. (The attorneys should be under oath, as I think that statement would be perjury. Attorney Rabin clearly meant every word and act.) The prosecutor asks that defense not use the word "embarrass." He agrees.

I think everyone in the courtroom has been traumatized by the defense attorney's badgering. His treatment of that young man was inhumane. But if it was a ploy, it worked: He has gotten Jason Hutson's testimony thrown out—and prevented any expert witness from stating an opinion on anything revealed in that testimony. This means that no expert witness will be able to speak to the fact that Dr. Klein saw two patients—Jason and his mother—in the room at the same time. That he made no examination of either. That both left with pain pills. In other words, the attorney for the defense was willing to do anything to win—regardless of the cost to the truth or to the witness he bullied.

The judge again comments on the length of the trial, asking, "How much longer is this trial going to take?"

> PROSECUTOR: Judge, I have no control over time. I did not think cross-examination would take two to three hours for some witnesses. And one was five hours.
>
> JUDGE: When is this going to end?
>
> PROSECUTOR: Judge, I have five witnesses left.
>
> JUDGE: You're losing your jurors. You think you're going to get through five witnesses on Tuesday?

DEFENSE (butter could have melted in his mouth): Judge I have always said I thought this case was going to take longer by a week. I would say honestly this week or the next. It's not like I'm trying to sabotage this case.

JUDGE: No one is saying anyone is trying to sabotage this case. Both of you need to figure this out. This case should have been finished today, September 4. Granted we had to cancel one day due to the possibility of the hurricane.

(As mentioned earlier, Monday, August 31, the West Palm Beach Courthouse was closed, due to reports that Hurricane Erika might hit Florida. And today, Friday, September 4, is the start of the Labor Day weekend; therefore, court will not be in session on Monday, September 7. The judge goes on to say some of these jurors have a conflict.

JUDGE: You knew that during jury selection some of these jurors are leaving for vacation at the end of next week.

DEFENSE [again, Eddie Haskell]: Judge, I've always contended that we should have picked alternates.

JUDGE: We do have two alternates.

DEFENSE: I contended that we might need more.

JUDGE: Not to me, you didn't say that.

DEFENSE: I said it to the assistant state attorney.

PROSECUTOR: Out of the five witnesses I have left, I know that two are going to be lengthy.

JUDGE: At this rate, you don't even know if you'll be done by the 18th. This is not your first rodeo. The two of you should have gotten together on this.

DEFENSE: I have two witnesses, and, of course, the big question—will my client testify?

JUDGE: No one is saying you can't try your cases.

I do not believe for a minute that the defense attorney's client, Dr. Klein, will be testifying. An administrative complaint was filed against Dr. Klein on October 24, 2012. That complaint involved patients other than those addressed in this trial. Subsequently, Dr. Klein voluntarily relinquished his license to practice medicine. The prosecutor cannot bring this up unless she is questioning Dr. Klein. There is no way on God's green earth that Dr. Klein will be sitting in that witness chair.

DAY TEN: TUESDAY, SEPTEMBER 8, 2015

When I enter the courtroom, the defense counsel and prosecutor are talking to the judge. The jury is not present.

PROSECUTOR: On the cross examination of Jeff George on August 26, 2015, at 2:30 p.m., Mr. Rabin started to question [Jeff George] about Dr. Klein. He talked to him about Dr. Klein being the most difficult doctor to get to increase the number of medications written. Mr. Rabin also stated that Dr. Klein discharged the most patients. The defense also made the statement that Dr. Klein had the most patients on Suboxone. The next day, with Theo Obermeyer, the same questions were presented. Both [Obermeyer and George] agreed that the patient log would be the best indicator.

PROSECUTOR, continued: Agent Wise was deposed eight times. During one deposition, the defense counsel addressed the records and the patient log. They reviewed every East Coast Pain patient—the type of injury they had, what doctor they saw, including those who saw multiple doctors. On August 6, 2014, [the defense attorney] brings a timeline to Jeff George. He brought up every bad move Jeff George committed. On October 6 or 7, Defense Attorney Rabin stated that he couldn't find his timeline in his computer. He did produce a pie chart.

PROSECUTOR, continued: It is the State's belief that he did receive both documents. A copy of the supplement shows it is attached to the very records that contained the pie chart. The State's position is that, on cross-examination, the statements made by Mr. Rabin are misleading to the jury. The defense stated that Dr. Klein was the most difficult doctor to get to increase amounts, had the most patients discharged from service, the most on Suboxone. The State's intent, when Agent Wise testifies, is that this evidence can be addressed.

DEFENSE: First of all, Your Honor, this is the first time I'm hearing this. Second of all, I did not open the door to these records. At no time did I ask [Jeff George and Theo Obermeyer] if they ever looked at the records. The charts are not admissible for several reasons. If they separated out discharged patients, Suboxone patients, it's an apple/orange. They're trying to back-door in something. They're trying to make something admissible. I merely asked their personal opinion.

PROSECUTION: The State is not seeking to admit the charts, merely to allow Detective Wise to testify to what he analyzed. Judge, the defense has known since June 3, 2014, that Detective Wise was going to testify. [Defense Attorney Rabin] had over a year to go over the patient records.

DEFENSE: I opened the door? Sounds like the State wants to impeach Jeff George's testimony.

There is a special place for defense attorney Rabin. He makes statements while questioning witnesses that he wants the jury to hear, truth or not. The prosecutor needs the detective to testify to prove the statements made by the defense were in fact not true. The defense's answer is to impeach another witness.

PROSECUTOR: Question by defense to George. "Isn't it true that when Dr. Klein found out they [two patients are named] were doctor shopping, he discharged them?" State pulled the files for the two patients, Your Honor. The first visit was with Dr. Bloom. The second patient was getting drugs on the street, and Dr. Bloom discharged them.

DEFENSE: This would be prejudicial, since we don't have the opportunity to look at the files. Another issue regarding Jason Hutson. I can declare a mistrial. I should give the instructions to the jury. This trial is infected with Jason Hutson. I respectfully move for a mistrial. I provided this to the state. If the report is not stricken from the record I file for a mistrial.

Records are stricken. Drug trafficking charges against Dr. Klein for drugs he prescribed to Jason Hutson are removed.

DETECTIVE WISE IS CALLED INTO THE COURTROOM (jury is not present)

Detective Wise is professional and able to speak to the subject of patient records being separated into files and spreadsheets.

> PROSECUTOR: Were you at one time employed by the DEA Task Force.
>
> DETECTIVE WISE: Yes. From 2008-2012.
>
> PROSECUTOR: Were you brought into the George brothers' empire, at East Coast Pain Clinic?
>
> DETECTIVE WISE: Yes.
>
> PROSECUTOR: Was a federal search warrant obtained?
>
> DETECTIVE WISE: Yes.
>
> PROSECUTOR: Did you have a chance to review the records?
>
> DETECTIVE WISE: Yes. I created a graph.
>
> PROSECUTOR: Your Honor, I'm showing this to the witness, what we discovered in discovery.
>
> DETECTIVE WISE: Yes, that is the spreadsheet.
>
> PROSECUTOR: What did you do with the information?

DETECTIVE WISE: We turned them over to the Palm Beach County analyst.

DEFENSE: Did you ever get a spreadsheet?

DETECTIVE WISE: Yes. I gave them to the prosecutor's office.

DEFENSE: Just for the record, Judge, I never saw that file.

PROSECUTOR: Did you take that spreadsheet and put it on a disk?

DETECTIVE WISE: Yes.

PROSECUTOR: If you put it side by side, the disk has all the information?

DETECTIVE WISE: Yes.

PROSECUTOR: Is the pie chart labeled East Coast Pain Clinic on a disk?

DETECTIVE WISE: Yes.

PROSECUTOR: Were these turned over at the same time?

PROSECUTOR: Your Honor, I have from the clerk's office that both of those were provided to the defense counsel.

DEFENSE: Your Honor, I don't have a discovery response from March 2009. I don't have any information regarding these persons. This is a discovery violation.

PROSECUTOR: Judge, counsel was given the pie chart. The witness has already testified that this was given at the same time. It automatically goes to the clerk's office and counsel. There is no reason why they wouldn't have it.

JUDGE: I don't find there was a violation. The information was provided. The disks were provided. He was deposed eight times. I don't find any issue for a violation. Bring the jury in.

The jury is brought back. Court is in session.

JUDGE TO THE JURY: The Fifth Amendment guarantees a witness can be questioned. It became apparent that Jason Hutson could not remember the past. You are to disregard the testimony of Jason Hutson.

PROSECUTOR: CALLS DETECTIVE WISE

PROSECUTOR: Detective Wise how are you employed?

DETECTIVE WISE: I have fourteen years with the Palm Beach Sheriff's Office.

Q. What are your responsibilities?

A. Aviation helicopter pilot. Before that, I was a police officer in West Virginia.

Q. What kind of degree do you hold?

A. Master's degree in public administration and a bachelor's degree in criminal justice.

Q. In your role in the narcotics division, how many arrests?

A. Hundreds, several hundreds.

Q. In how many of them were you the lead agent?

A. Hundreds.

Q. You wrote up seizures, search warrants. Ever have an opportunity to work on a multi task force?

A. Yes. The DEA.

Q. What was your role/assignment?

A. Ultimately, I investigated the case we're hearing today.

Q. Do you recall if the patient records were analyzed?

A. Yes. All the investigators were aware of what to look for.

Q. Did you make sure, as the case agent, that they were done correctly?

A. Yes. I went through every patient file.

Q. Once that was done, was East Coast Pain Clinic shut down and arrests made?

A. Yes.

Q. Agent, I'm going to show you what is going to be State Exhibit 23. Is this familiar?

A. Yes. This is what was given to me by the analyst.

Q. When you were reviewing the patient records, how many doctors worked at the clinic?

A. There were four.

Q. Are those also on the chart?

A. Yes.

They go through the number of patients that were discharged from the practice—very few. And which doctor saw them, etc. Looks like the defense is trying to indicate that Dr. Klein had more discharged patients than others, but he did not, really.

PROSECUTOR: No more questions, Your Honor.

DEFENSE: SAME WITNESS, DETECTIVE WISE

DEFENSE: We had an opportunity to meet several times. The investigation didn't start out of Miami right? It started in Kansas City, didn't it? DEA agents posed as patients online to order steroids right?

DETECTIVE WISE: Yes.

Q. Then Kansas notified the DEA here in Florida to assist them, right?

A. Yes.

Q. That fell to you. I don't know if you're low man on the totem pole. They found all kinds of stuff: steroids, time-share fraud, pain clinics.

Of course, the defense attorney is doing most of the talking, again. The witness can barely get an answer in.

DEFENSE: Just so we can be clear here, you were with the Palm Beach Sheriff's Office.

DETECTIVE WISE: Yes. My paycheck has always been with the Palm Beach Sheriff's Office.

Q. Now, part of all these compilations of files you gave to the analyst? And you believe them to be accurate?

A. Yes.

Q. Now, you said that Dr. Klein saw 376 patients. But Dr. Klein was there the longest, correct?

A. Yes.

Q. So the explanation is that he was there the longest.

A. Yes.

Q. Did he request prior medical records? I don't believe the prosecutor asked you about that. With respect to prior medical records of a patient, would that mean that they were requested or they were just found in the file?

Witness tries to answer and is cut off.

DEFENSE: That's not what I'm asking you. Dr. Klein 101. In that category, in that file, it would only be in the file if it was received, not whether it was requested or not?

DETECTIVE WISE: Yes.

Q. "Doctor shopping," that's a label. There was no central registry?

A. Correct.

Florida now has a central registry, the PDMP (Prescription Drug Monitoring Program). "Doctor shopping" refers to patients going from one doctor to another to get pills. The PDMP gives physicians a database through which to check whether a patient asking them for pills is also receiving pills from another doctor—possibly threatening the patient's wellbeing. (For instance, a patient seeing a psychiatrist for anxiety might not report to an emergency room doctor that they are on Xanax. Yet, the combination of Xanax and oxycodone, potentially prescribed for the pain resulting from an accident, is deadly.)

The PDMP became law in Florida in 2011. But there was great opposition to it. The opposition's claim was, as previously mentioned, that the PDMP was a HIPAA violation, that patients' privacy would be compromised by the PDMP. STOPPNow went to Tallahassee to support its passage. At this writing, October, 15, 2016, while Florida has implemented the PDMP, the American Medical Association and the Florida Medical Association only recommend that physicians use it. The State does not mandate that prescribers use it.

Yes. Although Florida is the epicenter of the prescription-pill epidemic responsible for so many deaths, politicians support only voluntary, not mandatory, use of the PDMP by prescribing physicians.

> DEFENSE: The only way for a doctor to know back then if the patient was doctor shopping is if they talked to the patient.
>
> DETECTIVE WISE: Yes, correct.
>
> Q. No central registry then. There is now. Doctors can no longer dispense. So things have changed.

Prior to 2010, doctors could dispense narcotics. And that they did. The intent of allowing dispensing of narcotics from doctors' offices was meant to help rural patients to obtain needed medications. Of course, in most of Florida, there is a pharmacy on every corner.

In 2010, though, legislation was enacted that stopped doctors from dispensing narcotics—a change that, no doubt, has saved (and will continue to save) many lives. However, there is a difference between "dispensing" and "prescribing." That difference has led to a misunderstanding that has been promoted, in part, by Florida Attorney General Pam Bondi, via the following statement, which she both displays on her website (as of this writing, October 15, 2016) and speaks about, publicly: *Florida's dubious distinction as the 'epicenter' of the nation's 'pill mill' epidemic was solidified in 2010 when DEA's Automation of Reports and Consolidated Orders System (ARCOS) reported that ninety-eight of the top 100 oxycodone dispensing physicians in the nation were located in Florida. Today, none of the top 100 dispensing physicians reside in Florida.*

While this may be factual, it also has misled many politicians to think the pill-mill problem in Florida is solved. However, what Attorney General Bondi leaves unsaid is this: While those ninety-eight top oxycodone dispensing doctors no longer dispense drugs, they have not (for the most part) lost their licenses to practice medicine and are still writing prescriptions. And, according to the CDC's 2014 report, deaths from prescription drugs are the highest they have ever been. The problem is nowhere near solved. In fact, despite the law to stop dispensing of narcotics from a doctor's office, passed in 2010, we have heard from businesses neighboring pill mills that people are still shooting up in pill-mill parking lots. This leads me to wonder if some pill-mill doctors are still willing to dispense to known clientele (so they are certain they are not dispensing to an undercover agent).

Back to the trial.

> DEFENSE: One other thing about the chart. I didn't ask you about the number of overdoses of each patient, total. The number attributed to Dr. Klein is one. During the time of your investigation, you did surveillance, and you reported nothing suspicious.
>
> DETECTIVE WISE: I don't know what you mean.

Good pickup by the witness. The defense attorney was trying to slip in, for the jury to hear, that there was nothing suspicious.

> DEFENSE: Did you see long lines?
>
> DETECTIVE WISE: No.
>
> Q. How many people did you see in the parking lot?
>
> A. Sometimes dozens.
>
> Q. You saw no lines?
>
> A. No.
>
> Q. Now, you don't know the people in the parking lot.
>
> A. Some we interviewed later.
>
> Q. Now you had two to three agents who went in undercover. Did you target doctors, or did you just see anyone?
>
> A. We saw anyone.

Q. Dr. Klein was not one of them.

A. Correct.

Q. Now, let's talk about three people you are familiar with: Jeff George, Theo Obermeyer, and Chris Hutson. There's a plea involved. Their time down to twelve-and-a-half years instead of seventy years. Now Jeff George. You were trying to find his money. He made millions, time-share fraud, etc. My question is that you know there are accounts overseas. Jeff George is going to have a significant amount of money when he gets out.

A. I believe he will.

Q. Jeff George also made many attempts to obstruct justice. Destroyed evidence. Jeff George offered people money to get him out of the country. Jeff George offered money to people to kill someone. Jeff George told people if anything happens to the clinic we blame the doctors. He was trying to kidnap someone named Eddy, and he was trying to destroy evidence. So this was one of the racketeering charges that was mentioned but not prosecuted. The State could have charged him, but part of the plea was that he wouldn't be charged with anything else. He could have been charged. Jeff George, John Eddy—threatened; put Uzi to ex-girlfriend's face when he thought she was cheating on him. He concealed a significant amount of assets, forged prescriptions, laundered money, time-share fraud, contacted owners with a scam to sell, made $10,000 a week. Then he started another business to provide legal counsel, and that was a fraud too. He was very accomplished at lying, correct?

A. Yes.

Q. During the time he was using steroids.

A. Yes.

Q. Over what period of time did you have contact?

A. 2010-2012.

Q. From your review of the patients' records, you are aware that Dr. Klein tried to wean people off of oxycodone, right?

A. No.

DEFENSE: May I approach.

The witness is shown a document.

DEFENSE: Do you believe he was trying to wean?

DETECTIVE WISE: No.

DEFENSE: You just read something where you did say it.

A. Yes.

DEFENSE: No more questions.

PROSECUTOR: ON REDIRECT, DETECTIVE WISE

PROSECUTOR: Who used the words "wean off" on page 11?

DEFENSE: Objection. Leading.

PROSECUTOR: Were they your words?

DETECTIVE WISE: No.

Q. When you agreed with what defense counsel was saying, that Dr. Klein actually was trying to wean off oxycodone, what did you mean? In your own words.

A. I guess if you look at what's there, they may have tried, but it never happened.

Q. Counsel asked you about approximately twenty-three acts that you discussed with George. Did he deny that he did those?

A. No.

Q. How did he act?

A. He was pretty arrogant.

Q. Did he seem to be proud of it?

A. Yes.

PROSECUTOR: No more questions, Your Honor.

DAY ELEVEN: WEDNESDAY, SEPTEMBER 9, 2015

Morning testimony edited out due to limited space.

I got back from lunch early. Behind me is a walkway that also has a bench. The second chair at the defense table, Michael R. Band, is pacing at the back of the courtroom. He states to those on that bench, in a humorous tone, that he wishes he had a tape of Rabin's cross-examination (referring to the judge asking Jason Hutson if he needed her to call 911). Mr. Band states he would sell it for CLE's (continuing legal education). I say nothing, but am seething. What I witnessed that day was no joking matter. The defense needed that testimony thrown out, as it was damning to their client, Dr. Klein. I can't take delight in it, and I am sickened that anyone else can.

THE STATE CALLS: GERRY JONES, D.O.

Dr. Jones is a young doctor who applied for a job fresh out of medical school and got it. As he testifies, it is obvious to this observer that he knows how fortunate he is to be sitting in the witness stand rather than standing trial.

PROSECUTOR: Can you state your credentials?

DR. JERRY JONES: I worked in urgent care for one year and five months.

Q. Can you tell us the difference between a D.O. and an M.D.?

A. Similar training. The D.O. does more manipulative treatment. I did my internship at Colombia University, in family practice.

Q. Did you ever serve in the ER?

A. Yes.

Q. Were you exposed to patients dealing with pain?

A. Yes.

Q. Did you work at East Coast Pain Clinic?

A. Yes from February 2009 to October 2009.

Q. How did you become aware of the position at East Coast?

A. One of the other students worked at another clinic, and he suggested I go to work there. Prior to that, I had been working with a podiatrist. He knew I was a med student and let me examine patients.

Q. In-house pharmacy?

A. Yes.

Q. What kind of medications?

A. Ultram, anti-inflammatory.

Q. Was it arranged to have an interview with East Coast Pain Clinic?

A. Yes. I met with Theo and Jeff George.

Q. How long did the interview last?

A. Very brief. Ten minutes, fifteen minutes, tops.

Q. Do you remember what you discussed?

A. Jeff was very quiet. Theo asked if I was comfortable writing prescriptions for pain medications.

Q. Did he mention what type of pain medications?

A. Yes, oxycodone.

Q. Were there any other type of drugs mentioned?

A. Yes, Xanax and Soma.

Q. Were there any other alternative forms of treatment discussed?

A. No.

Q. Any discussion about dosage levels?

A. Yes. 30 mg oxycodone is what they wanted written.

Q. Any indication of quantity?

A. Yes. 240.

Q. Prior to going there, did you know anything about the background of Theo, or Jeff?

A. Not at the time. I became aware later.

Q. Were you hired?

A. Yes.

Q. Any discussion about a dispensing license?

A. No. I didn't have one. I had to apply for it.

Q. When you started seeing patients, did you write prescriptions?

A. Yes.

Q. Were you only writing prescriptions, or did you offer anything else to the patients?

A. I tried to refer to neurology.

Q. What would happen?

A. Theo approached me and wasn't happy. We were losing patients.

Q. Did you maintain the quantity level that they wanted you to prescribe, 240?

A. Initially. When I tried to wean the amount, Theo would ask why I was decreasing the amounts of medications prescribed.

Q. While you were working there and treating patients, were you aware of a variation of treatment or all similar: oxycodone, Xanax, and Soma [muscle relaxer] prescribed for all the patients?

A. Pretty consistent.

Q. When you worked there, did you become aware of a shortage of oxycodone?

A. Yes.

Q. Was there an effect on the patients?

A. Yes.

Q. Was there a discussion?

A. I believe they talked about changing from oxycodone to Dilaudid. Ultimately it was up to Theo.

Theo, who has no medical training, but did once have a contractor's license.

PROSECUTOR: At some point did you start to prescribe different drugs?

DR. JONES: Yes.

Q. Were other drugs being ordered?

A. Dilaudid, Xanax, and Soma.

Q. Did you start making an inventory of drugs in your name?

A. There was a daily book, and you had to sign off on it. Theo would bring the forms for what he was going to order, and we would have to sign them.

Q. Would you tell Theo what drugs you wanted to order and what quantity?

DEFENSE: Objection.

The attorneys approach the bench. State repeats the question.

PROSECUTOR: Had you asked Theo to order those specific drugs?

DR. JONES: No.

Q. When East Coast switched to Dilaudid, was there any conversation, any measurement referred to about how patients receiving oxycodone should be converted to Dilaudid? How to convert?

A. I believe Dr. Klein had a thick green book on how to convert from one to the other.

Q. Were you familiar with the conversion?

A. I usually looked it up on the Internet, medical sources.

Q. Are they the same component?

A. When switching from one opioid to another, you want to back down twenty percent or so.

Q. Did you become aware of the death of Mr. Bartolucci?

A. Yes.

Q. Were you working that day?

Dr. Jones starts to cry. A short break is called. The witness is able to compose himself and take the stand once again.

PROSECUTOR: I'll take you back to where we left off. Conversions. Dr. Klein had a green book. There came a time that you became aware of the patient's death. At that time, did you have another discussion about the conversion that was used?

DR. JONES: I'm not sure.

Q. Did you know if Joseph Bartolucci had a file?

A. I believe so. Dr. Klein had received a letter from the BOM. He was writing a letter.

Q. Do you remember having a discussion about the conversion?

A. I believe he thought it was correct.

Q. Do you remember discussing the calculation upon learning about Dr. Klein's conversion? Did you have concerns about that? Did it appear that the calculation had been cut down?

A. I don't recall. I don't think so.

DEFENSE: Objection. Answer already given.

PROSECUTOR: What was your memory?

DR. JONES: I don't recall.

Q. But at the time, did you know that it should have been cut down?

A. Yes.

Q. Can oxycodone and hydromorphone be ordered equally one to one?

A. No.

Q. Were you making observations about the type of patients who were coming to the clinic?

A. Yes, some patients didn't seem like they should have been prescribed what they were being prescribed.

Q. Were you prescribing those as well?

A. Yes.

Q. Did there come a point in time that you decided to leave East Coast Pain Clinic?

A. Yes. I went on vacation to California and decided to go back to family medicine.

DEFENSE: SAME WITNESS, DR. JONES

DEFENSE: Dr. Jones, it would be fair to say that you are in an awkward position by being here?

DR. JONES: It's uncomfortable.

Q. You were questioned by the DEA, and you thought you were going to be charged?

A. Yes.

Q. When you started meeting with the federal prosecutor, you were terrified. You saw your whole career going up in smoke.

A. More than that.

Q. You were given immunity. Also on your mind, you could get reported to the board?

A. That's always a possibility.

Dr. Jones doesn't know that, in a great disservice to the public and to the doctors, the medical boards are doing nothing.

DEFENSE: The prosecutor asked you what type of drugs the podiatrist that you worked for ordered. You didn't mention any narcotics. Why?

DR. JONES: He prescribed a variety of medications.

Q. He was not limited to non-narcotics, right?

A. Right.

Q. The prosecutor asked a question about the patients you observed. You thought they were legitimate patients, right?

A. There were some who looked like they were there seeking pain medications.

Q. That was after you spoke to the federal prosecutor.

A. One time, there were three people outside, and I walked out there. I overheard them say, "Be careful. There's a snake in the grass." I told Dr. Klein that I wasn't going to see that patient. The other was to see Dr. Klein. Dr. Klein still saw them. He said, "I'll ask them about it."

Q. The reason you left was because of the DEA. Theo wanted you to see out of state patients. In fact, you were seeing out of state patients at another clinic, weren't you?

A. They had me work at another one of their pain clinics, yes.

Q. In fact, it was Dr. Klein who told you not to see out of state patients, and if they're coming from another state it has to be to get pills, correct?

A. I don't recall that conversation.

Q. Take a look at this and see if it refreshes your memory.

A. Yes, OK.

Q. Dr. Klein told you that it didn't make sense to him that they would drive all that way. You felt Dr. Klein was right about that, and you changed your position.

South Florida was known at the time as the OxyContin Express. People were driving down from as far as New York, Kentucky, and the Appalachian Trail to get pills. And they got them—as many as they wanted. Was Dr. Klein being cautious because out of state plates were starting to be observed and looked for by the DEA and law enforcement?

DEFENSE: The prosecutor asked you about the paper across the examining table in the room. No sinks. Do you remember seeing Purell?

What a joke. Really? Purell? Florence Nightingale must be turning over in her grave.

DEFENSE: The prosecutor asked you about Dilaudid 8 mg. And, in fact, you wrote prescriptions for that 8 mg of Dilaudid, correct?

DR. JONE: Yes.

Q. Dr. Klein had a target when prescribing.

A. Yes.

Q. He wanted to get to 180, correct?

A. Yes, I believe so.

Q. Oxycodone lasts four hours, so six pills a day equals 180 per month, right? By the way, you were writing higher? 240?

A. Yes.

Q. You were writing 8 mg Dilaudid.

A. Yes.

Q. Do you remember looking at the Dilaudid Dr. Klein prescribed?

A. Yes. I looked at it quickly.

Q. Quickly or slowly, you checked it right?

A. Yes.

Q. When you worked at East Coast Pain Clinic you never thought you did anything inappropriate.

A. Yes.

Q. Here is your deposition. Did he [Theo] ever get you to do something that you believed to be medically inappropriate?

A. No.

Q. Did he ever get you to do anything illegal?

A. I don't know.

Q. Now, obviously, when you're talking to the DEA agents and the federal prosecutors you had a baptism in criminally illegal. You have a totally different attitude now than you did then.

A. Certainly.

PROSECUTOR: ON REDIRECT, DR. JONES

PROSECUTOR: You were read a passage [from your deposition with the defense team].... What is it that you meant when you said at the time? What were you being shown?

The prosecutor is citing page 103 of Dr. Jones's deposition. The passage she references mentions that Dr. Jones was prescribing the same 8 mg of Dilaudid that Dr. Klein did. Dr. Jones was also prescribing oxycodone, and sometimes at even higher doses than Dr. Klein. This was a new doctor who went on the wrong interview. I really hope this is one of life's lessons for him, and that he can continue on to the career that was intended for him. He got lucky. I think he knows it.

DR. JONES: Just what they were prescribing.

Q. And who are "they"?

A. The other doctors.

Q. And do you know better now?

A. Absolutely.

Q. You mentioned the patients who were questionable. Do you know what Dr. Klein talked to them about?

A. No.

Q. Although Dr. Klein stated that he didn't want to see out of state patients, weren't they coming in?

A. Yes.

Q. Even though Dr. Klein said he was more comfortable with 180, are you aware that Dr. Klein was writing 200 and 240? Were warnings contained in the conversion literature?

A. Yes.

PROSECUTOR: No more questions.

THE STATE CALLS: DR. MARK RUBENSTEIN

As mentioned earlier in the text, I first met Dr. Mark Rubenstein at the Florida Board of Pharmacy Controlled Substance Standards Meeting held August 10, 2015. I attended the meeting to support the DEA. Doctor Rubinstein was invited to that meeting as a representative of the Florida Medical Association (FMA). He serves as both a delegate to the FMA and as an alternate delegate to the AMA and is Chairman of the FMA Council for Ethics and Judicial Affairs. As I concluded my statement to the pharmacy board, I asked for support from the FMA for the mandate of the PDMP and was given an affirmative nod. However, after the meeting, Dr. Rubenstein told me that the FMA and AMA would only *recommend* that doctors use the PDMP; they would not support *mandating* its use. His objection? Doctors could go to jail with such a mandate in place. And legislators do not want to sign their name to support a bill that would cost them the voting power of the FMA and the AMA. So the deaths continue.

Imagine my surprise, then, when he, Dr. Mark Rubenstein, walks into the courtroom to testify as an expert witness for the State—and, as we will learn, is making $750 an hour to do so! It seems everyone is making money from this epidemic, including this member of the board of ethics of the FMA. Yes, he is here to testify for the prosecution, however, the deaths will continue without much-needed change in our laws. We need the approval of the FMA and AMA in order for the deaths from the opiate epidemic to cease to rise each year. What we need are leaders who will not be intimidated by the FMA, AMA, nor the drug lobbyists.

PROSECUTOR: Doctor, tell the jury your credentials.

DR. RUBENSTEIN: I am a self-employed physician. I received my doctor of medicine from the State University of New York Health Science Center in Syracuse. I have attained board certification in three specialties, including physical medicine and rehabilitation, pain medicine, and electro-diagnostic medicine. I am a voluntary assistant professor of physical medicine and rehabilitation, as well as an assistant professor of medicine at the Miller School of Medicine at the University of Miami. I am also an affiliate assistant professor of biomedical science at Florida Atlantic University. I am chairman of the FMA Council for Ethics.

Q. After you reviewed the medical records, did you talk with me?

A. Yes.

Q. In your training and experience, are you familiar with the standards of care?

A. Yes. Opiates are just one form of treatment. There are other modalities to treat pain—physical therapy, chiropractor, massage therapy, exercise, to name a few. Pain should be individualized, with the least risk possible to the patient.

Q. Are there standards in place that require a physician to determine the appropriate history of a patient's pain problem?

A. Yes. If a new patient reports, "I've been taking [drugs] . . ." First of all, why are you seeing me now? If a patient has been on high doses of an opiate for a long time, wean them. Make modifications. A plan of care should be how to best optimize care for the patient. It's not one drug fits all.

Q. If an individual has been on oxycodone 30 mg from 180 to 240 a month, is there a way to determine if a patient should stay on that?

A. First of all oxycodone 30 mg puts a patient at a high risk for addiction. There are very few indications to take that many per month.

Q. Should a physician rely only on a trust factor between doctor and patient?

A. Pain is subjective. That's what drug addicts do. Lie, steal, that's what they do. My first reaction is addicted. I would look to see if I can help them change their life. If they say the only thing that works for me is oxycodone 30 mg to me, red flag.

Q. Is making an accurate diagnosis effective?

A. Absolutely. For instance, low back pain is a symptom—where is the pain coming from?

Q. How does a physician go about determining the reason?

A. Let's say they present with radiating neck pain. Is it adequate to simply tell them to bend over at the waist? Not at all. Range of motion [ROM] is only one part of a determination. A generic test does not justify high doses of medication.

Q. Are there procedures for calculating switching of medications? Opioid conversion factors? What risks are you concerned about?

A. Death. Respiratory distress is a real possibility. Does a patient necessarily need to be on another medication like Xanax if they don't need to be? They are both CNS [central nervous system] depressants.

Q. Oxycodone 30 mg 150 per month combined with 2 mg Xanax 60 per month—are there serious adverse effects?

A. There are very serious adverse effects, individually, and more so in combination.

Q. Is it important to discuss adverse effects?

A. We have to look for: Are they using it, or are they selling it? We have a huge problem in this state. With the higher doses of opiates, they will probably be constipated. Decreased intestinal motility is a side effect of the opiate.

Q. Are there considerations that must be taken into account when switching from one opiate to another?

A. Yes—cross tolerance. Just because you're tolerating one, doesn't mean you'll tolerate the other. There is a suggested calculation and how we start the patient. We start at a lower dose, then work our way up if necessary.

Q. So is it appropriate when taking 30 mg oxycodone 150 per month to switch to hydromorphone 8 mg 150 per month?

A. Absolutely not. The recommendation is no more than twenty-five to fifty percent of dose and then, depending on how it is tolerated, you may increase.

Q. Is that just a recommendation?

A. No. The published literature is always twenty-five to fifty percent of dosage to start. It is a question that is on the board exam that I have written.

Q. Have you had a chance to review the patient Alejandro Pina's records and do you have a recommendation? Did you reduce that to a report?

A. Yes. There is an MRI, CXR from St. Mary's hospital, a document from a place called CARP [a detox center in Palm Beach], and prescriptions. MRI disk bulging L1-L2 severe 2, 3, 4, 5 doesn't mean anything without a physical exam. Twenty percent of twenty year olds have bulging disks either on an MRI or a diagnostic image.

Q. Did the fact that the MRI was a year old mean anything significant?

A. More significant to me is that the patient was seeing another pain management doctor.

Q. After reviewing the file and a presentation of lower back pain, what is your opinion?

A. The first thing is that there was substandard record keeping. One: Initial visit was hand written. The patient history is illegible. Two: Complete physical that was not complete. Three: Hadn't obtained the medical records from the other pain management doctor. Four: Did not note that he read or commented on St. Mary's records in the file, where the patient admitted to using cocaine and going to rehab. The patient uses street drugs.

Q. Is there a fax date when East Coast received the records from St. Mary's?

A. February 12, 2009.

Q. When was Alejandro Pino's first visit to East Coast Pain Management?

A. January 29, 2009. Second visit, February 26, 2009 after receipt of those records.

Q. On notes by the physician, is there any discussion? On February 26, 2009, was he prescribed oxycodone, Xanax? Are any of those medications described in St. Mary's records regarding what he was detoxing from?

A. Roxi and Xanax. Progress note from February 26, 2009: Oxycodone 230 and Xanax 90. No reference as to why the patient would receive Xanax. Why is this patient on oxycodone and Xanax at all, with a history of drug abuse? Why not discuss detox? Standards of care would be to refer this patient to a rehabilitation center.

Q. What else can you tell us about February 26, 2009? On January 29, 2009, you had indicated he got oxycodone 240 and Xanax 90 and on February 26, 2009, oxycodone 230 in addition to Xanax 90?

A. It is not appropriate for anyone using street drugs to be prescribed these drugs. All highly addictive. Why he's on Xanax 2 mg very high dose—three times per day, 90 per month—is highly indicative of drug addiction. My opinion is that there was not a legitimate reason to prescribe these medications.

The patient that they are discussing, Alejandro Pino, received these medications *after* being granted custody of his children. The trial ended here for the day.

DAY TWELVE: THURSDAY, SEPTEMBER 10, 2015

PROSECUTOR RESUMES: SAME WITNESS, DR. MARK RUBENSTEIN

PROSECUTOR: Tell us about the value of a urine drug screen.

DR. RUBENSTEIN: There was none in Chris Hutson's file. We knew the patient had seen another doctor. No records were in the file. The only treatment in the file was high dose medications. No urine drug screen, which would have answered the question, is the patient compliant? Is he actually using the drugs?

Q. After review of the file do you have an opinion?

A. I could not justify the high doses of oxycodone in this case.

Q. Now, in the case of Joseph Bartolucci. Just let the jurors know what medical records you received?

A. I reviewed the whole file. They did receive records from Dr. W. Dr. W. was prescribing Percocet and prednisone [steroid]. Dr. W. had documented a physical exam.

Q. Any significance to the Percocet?

A. He was seeing another doctor that was prescribing a controlled substance, and he still saw Dr. Klein.

Q. Doctor, go ahead with your impression. What you found significant.

A. I reviewed the intake file. It explains the policies, charges, consents needed; there is correspondence, a complaint received against the doctor from the patient's mother.

Many mothers who have protested in front of pain clinics with STOPPNow previously went to a doctor who was prescribing opiates to their child and asked the doctor to stop prescribing them. These mothers told the doctors that their child was addicted to the drugs—to no effect. They ended up burying their child, and the doctors continued to prescribe, with their licenses intact.

DR. MARK RUBENSTEIN: In my review, despite the fact that they had records from another doctor who was treating the patient with Percocet, there were excessive amounts of oxycodone, Xanax, and Dilaudid prescribed for this patient. They are all drugs that affect the CNS. The patient had been put on Percocet for at least four weeks. And then Mr. Bartolucci was given a prescription from Dr. Klein in December for 15 mg of oxycodone, amount 150. Going from Percocet with 5 mg of oxycodone four times a day to oxycodone 15 mg five times a day—and up to six times a day because he wrote, "1 every 4 hours." Number one, that is aggressive, 90 mg per day. He told the patient to take one every four hours, very aggressive. Especially a twenty-four-year-old.

PROSECUTOR: Why do you say that?

A. Risk of addiction.

Q. What did you notice on the visit of January 29, 2009?

A. The prescription was changed to 30 mg, amount 120. He now doubled the dose of oxycodone from 15 mg to 30 mg. The prescription did not even tell the patient how often to take the medication.

Q. Is that required by the state?

A. Yes. A valid prescription must give instructions.

Q. Any physician note on January 29, 2009? Was there anything to justify the increase?

A. No. Doctor's note: "No job, pain unchanged, patient most likely took OxyContin from stepfather." I would have suggested that this patient go back to the surgeon. May need further tests. What is going on? Regarding the note that the patient took his stepfather's OxyContin—red flag.

Q. Any record regarding patient counsel?

A. No, and no referral for an epidural. Simply a note saying that the patient needs an epidural injection. My staff would have set up the appointment.

Q. On February 27, 2009, what medications did he receive?

A. Oxycodone 30 mg 150, take every four hours. Handwritten across the prescription was the word "void."

Q. What is the significance of that prescription?

A. 180 mg per day, if filled. There is a concern about the patient taking that much for non-malignant pain, non-palliative care.

Q. Are there concerns for a patient taking these medications?

A. Escalating pain that's not controlled. The only way I would use that much would be for an end-stage cancer or if a patient had acute pain [for a short time]. The patient was also prescribed Xanax 2 mg amount 15 and told to take half at night, rather than as needed.

Q. Is there a reason to prescribe a 2 mg tab if a physician wants the patient to take 1 mg?

DEFENSE: Objection. Leading.

JUDGE: Witness may answer.

DR. RUBENSTEIN: Sometimes, if insurance only covers the higher dose, or if they are out of a dosage. The patient was then prescribed Dilaudid 8 mg, 150, Xanax, Dilaudid and Nortriptyline—three different agents to depress. You just don't start a patient on Dilaudid 8 mg, but the three together puts the patient at a significant risk.

PROSECUTOR: Of what?

A. Death. Xanax, you don't use that on a twenty-four-year-old. Nortriptyline is another story. It is very appropriate, but you don't need both.

Q. When a physician practices pain management and ultimately provides medications, is there a treatment plan that should be on file?

A. Yes. Patients should be individualized. Evaluate what this patient needs. In a case like this, if the treatment is not working, why would you increase the medications? Why not try something else?

Q. Did you see any indication of this?

A. No. The only other note is a plan to follow up with neurology. I noted the lack of a physical exam, prescriptions in extreme high doses. Doctor should have realized this patient is drug seeking. One other caveat: the prescription is still in the file, voided. There is a bar code on there because . . .

DEFENSE: Objection, Your Honor. Barcode on their in-house pharmacy—that would be speculation! You don't know if he received it.

DR. RUBENSTEIN: Based on everything here, Dr. Klein used an aggressive and dangerous course of action.

PROSECUTOR: You've already indicated, which were outside of the standard of care.

A. Correct.

Q. Have you prescribed hydromorphone?

A. Yes.

Q. Under what conditions would you prescribe it?

DEFENSE: Objection. Relevance.

JUDGE: Witness allowed to answer.

DR. RUBENSTEIN: If a patient is not tolerating, sometimes I'll use rotation.

PROSECUTOR: How about oxycodone?

A. Very rare that I would order 30 mg oxycodone. Very rare that I would prescribe. I currently have no patients on oxycodone 30 mg. I wouldn't hesitate to use it for an end-stage cancer or palliative-care patient.

PROSECUTOR: No more questions, Your Honor.

SECOND CHAIR DEFENSE MICHAEL R. BAND: SAME WITNESS, DR. MARK RUBINSTEIN

DEFENSE: We've met on two occasions. January and March for depositions?

DR. RUBENSTEIN: Yes.

Q. Let's start with areas of your qualifications. You provided a CV to the state?

A. Yes.

Q. I had asked for it in January, and you said you were preparing one.

DEFENSE: I would like to put on record that I just got it today.

JUDGE: Would you like to review it?

DEFENSE: I don't want to stop questioning to review it.

JUDGE: OK. Then, let's move on.

DEFENSE: Can we approach?

They all go up to bench. We don't know what is discussed.

DEFENSE: Dr. Rubenstein, let me ask you a few questions about your CV. Subspecialty in pain medication. You're not an anesthesiologist?

DR. RUBENSTEIN: No.

Q. Have you ever had a fellowship in pain management?

A. No. They didn't have them when I was in medical school.

Q. You published some articles. How many?

A. Eight.

Q. Have you ever been invited to write a textbook?

A. I've been invited to write chapters in textbooks.

Q. Have any been published?

A. Not to my knowledge.

Q. What does "voluntary position" mean? What does "assistant affiliate" mean?

A. I was assigned to biomedical engineering to teach medical students.

Q. So you're not paid?

A. Right. I have my own practice. I volunteer to teach students.

Q. And your practice, physical medicine and rehab?

A. Yes, and pain management. Combination of orthopedic. It involves diagnostic and therapeutic.

Q. I think you testified you use low dose medications?

A. I use high dose too.

Q. Now high/low is subjective.

A. Yes, sir.

Q. In an article regarding high dose, in regard to consensus on what is a high dose and what is a low dose. Are you familiar with the article published in 2009? What constitutes a high dose?

A. That's one of those things that there are opinions and debates on.

Q. Recognize the journal?

A. Yes. It's something published by the American Pain Society.

Remember the senate investigation? A letter was sent to Purdue Pharma to answer questions based on a report from the *Milwaukee Journal Sentinel/Med Page Today* and Pro Publica revealing extensive ties between companies that manufacture and market opioids and non-profit organizations, such as the American Pain Foundation, the American Pain Society, the American Academy of Pain Medicine, the Federation of State Medical Boards, and the University of Wisconsin Pain and Policy Study Group.

DEFENSE: Let me show you what I'm referring to. Would you read this paragraph? The paragraph regarding guidelines. OK. This was published in February 2009 and, again, we're in September 2015. Every day, medicine is advancing?

DR. RUBENSTEIN: We hope so.

Q. In the lense [era] from 2009, they describe a consensus. A discussion to guide the practitioner. They describe a high dose as 200 mg daily. So if we're talking about oxycodone that's 135 mg per day.

A. Where did you get that 135 mg?

Q. Use your conversion table. The daily dose equivalent 135 mg of oxycodone and daily dose of Dilaudid 50 mg. I just want to be able to define terms you've used—"high dose."

A. I just want to state there are some articles, some literature that is highly controversial. There is tension in this community. It's not that I don't believe in opiates. I use them.

Q. In 2009, you gave expert witness testimony. This reflects that during a five-year period that you were hired by a lawyer to testify.

A. Yes.

Q. Some civil cases?

A. Yes.

Q. The vast majority of your cases are civil cases.

A. Yes.

Q. I believe you told Ms. Burns you appeared one to ten times. You appeared for federal court.

A. Yes.

Q. You know Ms. Burns? You called her Barb.

A. I have testified for the state, yes.

Q. Have you ever appeared for the defendant? You have never come to trial and sat in that chair and testified in criminal court for the defendant. If we do a rough break down, 150 cases in five years. That's thirty cases a year.

A. Correct.

Q. Let me ask you this: How much do you charge an hour?

A. $750/hr.

Q. State has their own rate.

A. Yes.

Q. And you agreed to abide by that?

A. Yes.

Q. How many hours do you have?

A. I've done many hours.

Q. Depositions are billable hours, testimony in court, review of the files.

A. There are many things that I haven't billed.

Q. When I deposed you and asked when you were first contacted, you weren't sure who you spoke to or how many hours you spent, but you were going to be receiving records.

A. Correct.

Q. December 22, 2010, notes you had a telephone conversation with Bill Frazier. You didn't know exactly what you were going to testify.

A. Yes. Ms. Burns came to my office once or twice. She reviewed the areas that I needed to testify.

Q. There are a number of items in your report that you don't know who gave you the information. The best way would be if you had written a note?

A. Yes.

Q. When you testify in a civil case, do you make billing notes? All the information you got came from the state attorney's office.

A. I've done investigation on statutes.

Q. But as far as the patient files that came from the state attorney?

A. Yes.

Q. Then you trust that the state attorney is giving you correct information?

A. I would assume a federal agency would provide me with correct information. I came to my own conclusion.

Q. You could have asked for other records if you wanted?

A. Yes.

Q. Physician experts reviewed the records right?

A. Yes.

Q. You could have ten experts review and all have different views.

A. Agreed.

Q. Let's say that you've been an expert 100 times. Generally speaking, there is an expert on the other side with a 180-degree different opinion.

A. Not always.

Q. You told me that an expert's opinion could be biased.

A. Agreed.

Q. You told me as an example ten radiologists could come up with different views.

A. Correct.

Q. For instance, H_2O is water.

A. That depends, too. You could get different answers on what chemical compositions are.

Q. The reason we give pain medication is to relieve pain.

A. Yes.

Q. Doctors are given a lot of leeway in how they treat pain.

But they're not supposed to kill the patients.

DR. RUBENSTEIN: Correct.

DEFENSE: The medical care that physicians prescribe is a judgment call?

A. Based on literature and standards.

Q. Facts were provided to you by the state. You're not sure when they came to you. You wrote in your report, for instance, that there were no exam tables.

A. My report says the exam rooms are limited and no exam table.

Q. So someone from the state attorney's office told you that.

A. Yes.

Witness shown exhibit 50, a picture of a room in the clinic.

DEFENSE: Does there appear to be an exam table?

DR. RUBENSTEIN: Yes.

Q. So that fact of information that was given to you and in your report is incorrect. The state attorney told you there was a limited time to examine patients. That's something that was relayed to you. Did you interview any of the patients?

A. No. Nothing I've just heard would change my opinion.

Q. You never met Mr. Bartolucci?

A. Correct.

Q. You weren't present at his exam?

A. Correct.

Q. You weren't present at his exam, nor did you speak to his other doctors. Did you speak to Chris Hutson?

A. No.

Q. Did you speak to Alejandro Pino?

A. No.

Q. People at the state attorney's office told you these things. They provided your primary source of information. The patient would give you a better view right?

A. Correct.

Q. Best example would have been if you could've performed the exam on them.

A. If you had a live patient. There would have been someone who could have answered that. [The defense attorney did not like the implication of that answer]. You asked the question, and I answered it.

Q. Excuse me, are you the lawyer?

The defense attorney is getting a little testy.

DEFENSE: We've had many people testify over these few weeks. Do you know if Chris Hutson is a cooperating witness?

DR. RUBENSTEIN: I'll defer to you.

Q. Mr. Hutson testified that he is receiving no benefit from his testimony. That he was doctor shopping. That he provided a fake MRI. That he over expressed his pain. He stated that Dr. Klein went over questions on the form and asked his own questions. And Dr. Klein decreased his prescriptions from 240 to 210. That Dr. Klein asked more questions at the second visit. On cross exam he admitted that he was a successful liar. He saw five doctors at three clinics. How did he learn to doctor shop? He had a professor. Have you ever heard of Jeff George?

A. Yes.

Q. Jeff George told him that Dr. Klein was straight. Dr. Klein was fooled by him. He remembers him using a stethoscope, checking reflexes. He remembers that he asked for 240 oxycodone. He knew how to play a part. He enjoyed his role. He employed some truth, a bike accident. He faked nausea. You mentioned urinalysis. He was given a urinalysis. It didn't come up with anything.

If the urinalysis didn't show anything, that means he wasn't taking the drugs, so was he selling them? The doctor on the stand, Mark Rubenstein, should have pointed that out. Of course, he was already accused of being a lawyer, and he wasn't really asked a question.

DEFENSE: He said pain was eight out of ten. Dr. Klein said, "You need to see a neck specialist." Dr. Klein said, "I'm weaning you." Did the State share that with you?

DR. RUBENSTEIN: We're not allowed to talk about the trial.

Q. Everything you're talking about was in the trial. They could have shared that with you as an expert, and they didn't.

A. Well, many of the patients at East Coast were doctor shopping.

DEFENSE: Judge, I have a motion.

They all approach the bench. We aren't privy to what is discussed. But my guess is the defense didn't like the unsolicited input from Dr. Rubenstein.

DEFENSE: Let's discuss Alejandro Pino. Assume he was in a very serious car accident. He was in the hospital for a month and a half. He brought in his own MRI. He said he walked in there and said it looked like a regular doctor's office. He reported tingling. He was a chef for Donald Trump. Now assume, on cross exam, he said he had a poor recollection in 2009. He received immunity from the State for doctor shopping, by the way. Dr. Klein said I'm going to cut you off of oxycodone. You know who Donald Trump is, right?

DR. RUBENSTEIN: Yes.

DEFENSE: Donald Trump is a very demanding guy.

DR. MARK RUBENSTIEN: Speculation.

DEFENSE: Again, are you the lawyer?

This is turning into a fun day.

DEFENSE: Now, nobody on Donald Trump's staff knew he was on drugs.

PROSECUTION: Objection, Your Honor. Speculation.

DEFENSE: [Alejandro Pino] went to CARP. He said he went to CARP to get his children back. Dr. Klein told him, at that time, he wanted to keep close scrutiny on him. The accident pinned him into the car. Did the state attorney's office give you any of the patient facts?

DR. RUBENSTEIN: Only what I saw in the medical records.

DEFENSE: You also indicated that you reviewed statutes that helped in forming your opinion. During the course of my deposition of you, you looked at the standards set by the BOM in 2003 and the fact that they changed a bit in 2010. Anywhere in those standards where there is any information regarding the second exam?

DR. RUBENSTEIN: The physician is required to keep accurate records of medical treatments.

DEFENSE: Objection, Your Honor. The witness is giving an improper editorial remark. I didn't hear an answer to the question I asked. You also stated that you looked at DOH records. They are the administrators for the BOM and the Board of Pharmacy, are they not? And they conduct an investigation. You're familiar?

DR. RUBENSTEIN: I am an expert.

DEFENSE: They receive a complaint; probable cause panel is assembled; a decision is made to get records. They issue a subpoena, do they not?

A. Yes.

Q. The state attorney's office gave you the subpoena, so that may aid you in rendering your opinion.

A. I've reviewed it.

Q. Then DOH contacts someone like you to deliver an opinion. That opinion goes to about fourteen other doctors and two lay people to make a decision.

A. I don't know how many people, but it is reviewed.

Q. There was a subpoena provided to you from the state attorney. They never gave you this report that the DOH panel found no probable cause. This was never shown to you?

A. Correct.

That's a big one for the defense. Too bad [Dr. Rubenstein] couldn't chime in that there was another complaint, and Dr. Klein relinquished his license. I, myself, have written to the State of Florida letting them know that there should be audits of the DOH and BOM decisions, all of which has fallen on deaf ears.

DEFENSE: Now you testified that Xanax 1 mg at night was a high dose, is that correct? Have you ever heard of Dr. Goldberger, toxicologist? He said that dose was OK. Did the State share that with you? You're familiar with the conversion of oxycodone to Dilaudid. You're board certified, correct?

DR. RUBENSTEIN: Correct.

Q. That involves sitting for an exam?

A. Yes.

Q. The patient's report of pain is a starting point.

A. Yes, typically.

Q. In your office do you have a polygraph machine?

A. No.

Q. Have you hired a private investigator?

A. I have in worker's comp cases, yes.

Q. Certainly, you examine the patient and look for signs that they are not telling the truth. And you look at their record, and it is subject to interpretation?

A. Correct.

Q. Physicians exercise judgment every day. There is a Patient Bill of Rights. Patient also has certain obligations to the provider.

A. I'm not sure I can speak of Patient Bill of Rights.

Q. So you know we're not making this up. Is this the Florida statute?

A. Yes.

Q. Again, the patient is supposed to provide complete and accurate information.

A. Yes.

Q. The patient is supposed to tell you about past medications.

A. If not, ask.

Q. They are supposed to tell you about past hospitalizations?

A. Again, sir, ask.

Q. They are supposed to follow the treatment plan.

A. Yes.

Q. The patient/doctor relationship is somewhat unique. You looked confused. Let me help you out. Anything shared with the rabbi, wife, even the state attorney, we can't get that information. So a patient can be confident when sharing information.

A. When a patient is drug seeking, it's my job to be the polygraph machine.

Q. There is a mutual obligation. Information that is provided should be truthful so we can walk this path together. Let me go through some of your testimony. It's generally a good thing to wean a patient from oxycodone. You want them on the lowest dose. You talked about red flags. Mr. Bartolucci reported he tried his stepfather's oxycodone.

A. Yes.

Q. History of psychological illness. Does that mean you would never prescribe opiates?

A. No.

Q. Let's talk about Mr. Pino. Three visits to Dr. Klein.

A. Correct.

Q. There's an indication from a fax that the patient came in December. But you don't know when it was placed in the file. There was a whole discussion about templates. A lot of facilities use templates.

A. Yes.

The use of a template is not the problem. A template is simply a list of predetermined questions on a patient's chart. The practitioner completing the assessment simply places a checkmark in the correct box (for example: *Lungs clear*, checkmark). It's the amount of medications prescribed that is the problem.

DEFENSE: Do you have your own shorthand?

DR. RUBENSTEIN: My notes are all transcribed.

Q. Pain is subjective.

A. Yes.

Q. Even as you sit here today, you can't draw blood and determine how much pain a patient is in?

A. Correct.

Q. In your discussion of Mr. Bartolucci and the amount of medication, I think in December, oxycodone 15 mg, quantity 150.

A. Correct.

Q. Depending on how you want to skew, five times a day would be 75 mg per day, or six times would be 90 mg per day.

A. The prescription was written, "Take every four hours."

Q. Wouldn't they be sleeping?

A. Sometimes they do wake up.

Q. Wouldn't the patient run out?

A. They could.

Q. So the correct interpretation is 70 mg per day.

A. I'm just interpreting from what is written.

Q. Now, you also indicated that you couldn't understand why the dose was increased. Because part of the note said, "Condition unchanged".

Read the whole sentence [from the document], "Perhaps increase in severity."

A. I'm troubled by . . .

Q. I didn't ask you if you're troubled. I asked does it say that? Turn back to the first progress note. Discussion about analgesia. "What is the pain level?" "Five to eight." "Does the current treatment give relief in your life, Mr. Bartolucci?" "No."

A. If I felt that a drug was indicated, and if I may answer, his pain levels had actually gone down. Why would I increase the medications?

Q. But he also says, "I don't have as bad a pain, but I'm not able to function." Also on 2/27 Nortriptyline. That is an adjunct medication, correct?

A. Correct.

Q. Is there any indication that he filled that?

A. There's a copy in the file. The original is missing; it has a barcode. It may have been filled.

Q. Did you inquire of Ms. Burns or Detective Frazier if the script from February 27, 2009, was filled?

A. I did inquire. They said it hadn't been.

Q. Then, as you sit here today, you knew it hadn't been filled, yet you indicated maybe it was. No further questions.

PROSECUTOR: ON REDIRECT, DR. RUBENSTEIN

PROSECUTOR: I'm going to start where we left off. Does it matter whether the prescription was filled or, for that matter, even if it was written?

DR. RUBENSTEIN: No.

Q. Even though doctors are given leeway, must they also comply to the standards in place?

A. Yes.

Q. Chris Hutson, all the lies, did that have any basis?

A. The real issue is the physician. The physician must look for drug seeking patients.

Q. Mr. Pino said that Dr. Klein took good notes.

A. The records speak for themselves.

The prosecutor also went through the standard-of-care questions being followed. Medical personnel are all familiar with the standard of care for any treatment rendered. In nursing, for example, the standard of care when placing a feeding tube is to check placement before using the tube to feed; caution must be taken due to the fact that the tube could be in the lungs. One must follow the standard of care to preserve one's license and, more importantly, to ensure safety of the patient.

The defense objected throughout.

> PROSECUTOR: As to the DOH, you were asked if you'd seen the investigative file?
>
> DR. RUBENSTEIN: Correct.
>
> Q. In your opinion when DOH . . .
>
> DEFENSE: Objection. Speculation.
>
> PROSECUTOR: If the report had been done after 2009, do you know if DOH would have had any or all of the State's investigation?
>
> DEFENSE: Objection. The witness is not allowed to answer.

PROSECUTOR: Previously, when you had answered questions during the deposition, you had spoken about Xanax in combination with other drugs. Multiple drugs.

DR. RUBENSTEIN: There are lower doses of Xanax. There is also no documentation why the patient was on that medication.

AT 2:45 P.M. THE STATE ANNOUNCES THAT THE STATE RESTS.

After break, before the jury returns, the defense team tries to get the judge to throw out some counts, saying that the State had not brought up the fact that the standards of care had not been followed for that particular case. This explains why the State asked the expert witness about the standards of care over and over. The judge informs the attorneys that she kept her own notes, and it was covered. They continue to go back and forth about several issues. The defense, in the end, states that the State failed to provide toxicology lab, and he is asking for a mistrial.

Sore loser.

JUDGE, TO THE DEFENDANT: Mr. Klein, you have the right to testify. I'd like for you to have that conversation with your lawyer. You do have the right to testify.

As mentioned earlier, the jury doesn't know that Dr. Klein has voluntary relinquished his license to practice medicine as the result of an administrative complaint filed regarding five patients treated by Dr. Klein. (That's five patients *in addition* to the four patients' treatment under scrutiny in this current trial—Chris Hutson, Jason Hutson, Alejandro Pino, and the deceased, Joseph Bartolucci.) None of this has been brought out in the trial. However, if Dr. Klein were to testify, the prosecutor could bring this to light.

THE DEFENSE PRESENTS THEIR CASE

DEFENSE CALLS: DR. CAROL WARFIELD, M.D.

Each side has their expert witness to bring home their side of the story. This must be confusing for the jury. That is all I have to say about Dr. Warfield.

DEFENSE: Please tell the jury about yourself.

DR WARFIELD: Profession, physician and pain management specialist. Further training in pain management, but most commonly anesthesia, but other specialties also. I started pain management at Harvard. I was the director for two years. My career has essentially been in pain management.

DEFENSE: State your opinion. Was Dr. Klein working as a legitimate pain doctor?

A. Yes.

Q. Board certified?

A. Yes, anesthesiology. Diplomat of Board of Pain Medicine. I put together a sub-specialty of pain management. Pain medicine became a board specialty. I have a number of academic appointments as well. I am a full time full professor at Harvard. Endowed professor. I was appointed to be on the FDA. I was actually on the committee that approved some of these opiates.

I would not be proud of that.

DR. WARFIELD: I was part of the International Conference on Opiates at Harvard. If someone wants to be board certified, they have to complete a fellowship. I served on the American Pain Society and was on the Board of the American Academy of Pain Medicine.

DEFENSE: You've written approximately thirty peer reviewed articles, as well as books.

A. I've written three textbooks.

Q. Are your books used in medical schools?

A. Yes, worldwide. I travel giving lectures. The clinic has a new name. The clinic at Harvard, they named it after me.

Q. You were treating with opioids?

A. Yes.

Q. They are FDA approved?

A. Yes. The pain is what the patient tells you it is. You rely on what the patient tells you.

Q. Have you had patients for longer than three months?

A. I've had patients for years.

Q. The pain medications that were used by Dr. Klein, are they the type of medications used by doctors?

A. Yes.

Q. You were actually in the courtroom when Dr. Rubenstein testified.

A. Yes.

Q. He spoke about the divide. Can you explain?

A. We all know opioids work. They have been around for years. We've never come up with a drug better than these. When I was a resident, we didn't use these drugs. In 1990 there was a big movement to treat chronic pain, not just cancer. People were over concerned. No one is denying they are addictive.

They, the drug companies and some doctors who wrote textbooks and spoke on behalf of the drug companies, absolutely were denying that—until they got caught.

DR. WARFIELD: There are two groups of doctors: One: Why are we allowing these people to suffer? Two: Some who believe we shouldn't use even for cancer patients. Some won't prescribe because they're afraid they're going to be indicted. So people are suffering. Most doctors are in the middle.

DEFENSE: Is Xanax used with oxycodone?

A. Yes, very common.

Common, but deadly. The CDC Guidelines published March 2016 state: *Clinicians should avoid prescribing opioid pain medication and benzodiazepines concurrently, whenever possible.* FDA Commissioner Robert Califf, M.D., also issued a strong warning. On August 31, 2016, he said, *It is nothing short of a public health crisis when you see a substantial increase of avoidable overdose and death related to two widely used drug classes being taken together.* The drugs he is warning against using together are opioids and benzodiazepines. Oxycodone and heroin are opioids; Xanax is a benzodiazepine.

DEFENSE: You've heard about some of the numbers, 30 mg quantity 150. Is that a high dose?

DR. WARFIELD: I would not have called this a high dose.

Q. The Dilaudid 8 mg 40 mg per day?

A. That's not a high dose, considering what he was taking. There's a lot of individual variation in what dose will work for each patient.

Q. If a patient has pain and also anxiety?

A. Yes, they can be combined, oxycodone and Xanax. Almost all my patients are on pain medications and anti-depressants. The dose he was prescribed would not have caused any problems. He would have had to have taken something else.

Q. Do you review other records?

A. I supervise 200 doctors. I work on peer reviews. So in my experience I review many records.

Q. How does Dr. Klein compare?

PROSECUTION: Objection.

All approach the bench.

DEFENSE: In regard to Dr. Klein and his three patients whose records you reviewed.

PROSECUTION: Same objection.

JUDGE: Overruled.

DR. WARFIELD: The records, what they contained, were usual. I think they were complete.

DEFENSE: Did they provide you with enough information to render an opinion?

A. Yes.

Q. You had an opportunity to review the file for Mr. Hutson, Mr. Bartolucci. Do you recall reviewing Mr. Bartolucci's file?

A. Yes.

Q. Did Dr. Klein treat Mr. Bartolucci?

A. Absolutely.

Q. Do you have an opinion whether those prescriptions were appropriate?

A. Yes. There was nothing there that would indicate that Dr. Klein wasn't acting in good faith. He was working in his office, doing physical exams, using MRI's. There's not just one way, and if you don't do it, you're a criminal. There are different medical practices.

Q. Now, urine drug screening.

A. Some doctors use them, and some don't use them at all. In 2009 there were no regulations in place to use drug screening. If you have a drug addict, they have become very good at fooling the system. They drink a lot of water. One can go on the Internet and buy something that they can inject someone else's urine into their bladder. So lots of doctors don't use them.

Q. After the initial exam, do you repeat a physical exam on the second visit?

A. You do a physical exam when you want to. No requirement that you must do a physical exam.

DEFENSE: No more questions.

PROSECUTOR: SAME WITNESS, DR. CAROL WARFIELD

PROSECUTOR: Regarding your textbook, you testified that you wrote them. Actually, you edited them.

DR. WARFIELD: Yes, I edited them. I would ask specific colleagues, like cancer specialists to write that particular chapter, and then I would edit them. It may have been that I wrote the first edition and then let my fellow, junior to me, write a chapter to give them experience. I would decide we need a book, and I would go to other disciplines. They would write and give it to me, and I would edit. I trained a lot of people over thirty years. Many opened pain clinics.

On the other hand, I have closed some down.

PROSECUTOR: Another chapter that you co-authored has three authors. Do you know how much you contributed?

DR. WARFIELD: I would have written the original edition, and then thirteen years later I would have asked people to update it. This is how we do things in academic medicine. It's to help train them.

Q. Do you know what specific universities are using these textbooks?

A. I've been told by McGraw Hill that it is the most used textbook.

Q. What is your rate?

A. I charge $500 per hour to review records and $750 per hour to testify.

PROSECUTOR: No more questions.

Court adjourns.

DAY THIRTEEN: FRIDAY, SEPTEMBER 11, 2015

Court is scheduled to start at 8:30 a.m. The defendant, Dr. Klein, is not here. They call downstairs and find he is going through security. He arrives at 8:42 a.m.

JUDGE: Is Dr. Klein testifying?

DEFENSE: No.

JUDGE: It's your decision, after speaking with your attorneys?

DR. KLEIN: Yes.

Just as I thought. The defense does not want it revealed that Dr. Klein voluntarily relinquished his license to practice medicine. The defense was successful earlier in revealing that the DOH found no grounds to discipline Dr. Klein regarding the complaint filed on behalf of Joseph Bartolucci. That is all the defense wants the jury to know.

Jury is brought into the courtroom at 9:05 a.m.

DEFENSE CALLS: DR. MARK GERBER

I found Dr. Mark Gerber to be professional. Dr. Gerber was asked by the DOH to review the complaint against Dr. Klein, which was filed by Mrs. Bartolucci. But a complaint should not have to be made against a doctor by a grieving parent. The State is aware of high-prescribing doctors. They are able to tally, by the DEA number, every prescription that is written. Yet the DEA, the MQA (Medical Quality Assurance), and the BOM have failed to protect the people of our state. I have requested meetings with the Florida Surgeon General and the MQA. As mentioned previously, I have also requested audits of decisions made by the MQA and BOM. But the deaths continue.

DEFENSE: Please tell the jury a little about yourself.

DR. GERBER: I am a physician specializing in physical medicine and pain. I treat acute and chronic pain. I see a lot of post-op patients. Many of my referrals come from hospitals.

Q. You work in Orlando. You moved to Florida after completing your residency in 1996. Board certified. Sub-specialty pain. You have also served as an expert for the Board of Medicine.

A. I've reviewed fifty to 100 cases.

Q. When you serve for BOM/DOH who hires you?

A. The DOH.

Q. You're not hired by a defendant?

A. No.

Q. Let's talk about your career in pain management. Are you currently working in the field of pain?

A. Yes.

Q. You actually know Dr. Rubenstein?

A. Yes.

Q. Pain is a disease.

A. Yes.

Q. Do you treat with oxycodone, Dilaudid?

A. Yes.

Q. There are tools that are available now that weren't available then.

A. The PDMP is now available, so you can check.

As previously noted, in Florida, the use of the PDMP is not mandatory for prescribers. Most do not use the database prior to writing a prescription for a narcotic. I have been unsuccessful, thus far, trying to gain support from our Florida legislators to make use of the PDMP mandatory, nor could I get support from the FMA (Florida Medical Association), despite the increasing deaths from opiates. To make matters worse, Florida just passed into law that nurse practitioners and physician assistants can now write prescriptions for narcotics without doctor oversight.

DEFENSE: You were asked by the DOH to review the file of Mr. Bartolucci?

DR. GERBER: Yes.

Q. The complaint was made by the patient's mother.

A. Yes.

Q. Now, you prescribe oxycodone?

A. Yes.

Q. Is it common for patients in pain to suffer from anxiety?

A. Yes.

Q. In regard to your review of the file for Mr. Bartolucci, you received his file from East Coast Pain Clinic?

A. Yes.

Q. Now, Dr. Klein is not perfect, right?

A. Right.

Q. Is anyone perfect?

A. No.

Q. How does Dr. Klein compare to other doctors you've reviewed?

A. Average.

Q. You know about the Patient Bill of Rights?

A. Yes.

Q. The patient has a responsibility to be candid with you, not to hide facts from you.

A. Yes.

Q. There is a primary focus of trust. That is so you can make a value judgment?

A. Yes.

Q. Was there any indication that Mr. Bartolucci had been in treatment?

A. No.

Q. Would that have affected your patient care?

A. Yes.

Dr. Klein's patient Alejandro Pino had been in treatment. But that didn't make a difference in the prescriptions he walked out with.

DEFENSE: Now, you have served as an expert for DOH/BOM?

DR. GERBER: Yes.

Q. We've all heard that doctors stick together. Tell us about your findings.

A. About twenty to twenty-five percent of the doctors did nothing wrong. Sometimes there are bad outcomes, and it's not the doctor's fault.

I would say that most doctors do care about the treatment and care of their patients. But what we are seeing, with the opiate oxycodone, is an easy way for doctors to use their license for greed. It is too easy, too tempting. Between 2007 and 2010, the timeframe under consideration, there were no consequences for opiate prescribers. It is a legal drug. It was very easy for these doctors to rationalize their actions—for half a million dollars a year. As for those who were dying? Well, it was their own fault. Not the doctors'. Their attitude: "I'm well educated; I'm held in high esteem. I have a license."

DEFENSE: Did you see his conversion?

DR. GERBER: Yes. Nothing was wrong.

Q. You even said it was conservative.

A. Yes.

DEFENSE: No further questions.

PROSECUTOR: SAME WITNESS, DR. GERBER

PROSECUTOR: Back in July 2009, the DOH sent you the file, and about a week later you wrote a letter?

DR. GERBER: Yes.

Q. Do you have the August 2009 letter? Isn't it a fact that you wrote, "Inappropriate"?

A. I'm sorry. That was a typo. I corrected it to the attorney.

Q. Didn't you also write that the handwriting was not clear, and there wasn't a treatment plan? You also said that you would not have prescribed that high a dose to a young person. Are you aware that Mr. Bartolucci was twenty-four years old?

A. Yes. My overall summary at the end is that [Dr. Klein] was following the standard of care.

Q. For this case you reviewed no other cases or patients of East Coast Pain?

A. No.

Q. Tell me about your practice. Do you have other employees?

A. Yes, five full time employees. Nurse, physician assistants.

Q. Does your practice take insurance?

DEFENSE: Objection.

JUDGE: Overruled.

DR. GERBER: Yes.

The pill mills are all cash only.

PROSECUTOR: Do you see that all of these patients paid $150 in cash and up to $500 for prescriptions?

DR. GERBER: I was not a dispensing physician. The goal is to treat patients with the least amount of medications as possible to relieve pain. I try other modalities if they don't work. I treat with medications.

Q. Do you give Percocet 5 mg?

A. Yes.

Q. So if I'm taking 30 mg oxycodone, that's six times the dose, compared to the Percocet. Do you ever consult with nonmedical people about what you're going to prescribe?

A. No.

Q. Would you ask a nonmedical person about the amount you are going to prescribe? For instance, quantity 180 oxycodone?

A. No.

Q. In August 2009, your days were filled. You have your own practice. You had no time to go down to East Coast Pain Clinic and see what they were doing, right? Do you know that they were closed down in March of 2009?

DEFENSE: Objection.

All approach the bench.

DR. GERBER: I know nothing about the practice.

PROSECUTOR: Now, oxycodone 30 mg, pretty potent stuff?

A. Yes.

Q. Now would you take an eighteen-year-old off the street and give him 30 mg oxycodone?

A. No. It could kill them.

DEFENSE: Objection.

To the bench.

PROSECUTOR: Oxycodone 30 mg every four hours, that could kill him, right?

DR. GERBER: Yes. If he is opiate naive [not used to the drug].

Oxycodone is such a highly addictive drug that many relapse after being clean for a time. However, once clean, they may no longer have the tolerance to the drug they once did—and when they take the drug again, many die.

PROSECUTOR: In your letter August 2009, you indicated that Dr. Klein's treatment plan was not noted.

DR. GERBER: It was hard to read, but overall I got the idea of what he was doing.

Q. Let's look at the February 27, 2009, progress note: "Activity of daily living adverse events, none." How many years have you been prescribing oxycodone?

A. Many years.

Q. Read this note to the jury [shows document to witness].

A. "Pain is unchanged. Patient took OxyContin from his stepfather. Patient liked it. Counseled." It's hard to read. I assume that the patient was getting OxyContin from his stepfather.

Q. Is that a red flag?

A. Yes. There's a lot of thought that should go into this. You may want to wean them or discharge the patient. Patient did say that with the oxycodone he was seeing improvement. It's helping. Could be he had a substance abuse problem (taking the OxyContin). Looks like he was considering an epidural. [Dr. Klein] counseled the patient. Like I said, the care wasn't perfect, but it was treatment.

Q. Now, the doctor Mr. Bartolucci was seeing before he saw Dr. Klein was not prescribing benzodiazepines with the opiate. Can you explain to the jury what effect that particular treatment can have?

A. It can cause respiratory depression, but he was on a low dose. The doctor must be aware of that. The dose he was prescribing was small. Yes, the crisis in Florida was from using the combination of benzodiazepines with the opiate. Those were higher doses.

Q. What is the highest Alprazolam (Xanax, benzodiazepine) that you know of?

A. Well, the 2 mg tablet is the highest.

PROSECUTION: No more questions.

DEFENSE: ON REDIRECT, DR. GERBER

DEFENSE: The dose of Xanax, you said that did not alarm you. You mentioned the crisis in Florida? 2 mg four times a day that was being dispensed at those clinics, and the combination was a problem. Again 1 mg dose at night does not concern you?

DR. GERBER: No.

Q. The prosecution talked about a hypothetical eighteen-year-old. Let's talk about Joseph Bartolucci. Was he opiate naive?

A. No.

Q. The red flag that the prosecution brought up. Mr. Bartolucci was honest. Does that mean that you stop treatment?

A. No. I encounter it a lot.

DEFENSE: Defense rests.

STATE CLOSING ARGUMENT: ASSISTANT STATE ATTORNEY BARBARA BURNS

It's been a long trial, exhausting, but a very important trial. It's the State's burden to prove beyond a reasonable doubt. You've heard a lot of testimony. Dr. Carol Warfield tried to educate you on what she thinks the law should be. It's about the law this judge read to you. Some of the instructions pertained to the patient's responsibilities. In order for this to apply, they would have to have been patients. These were not patients, though; they were drug seeking.

Theo Obermeyer admitted that he made the label, "customers." Jeff George talked about his business model. What they were trying to attract to the business. We found a website that attracted patients seeking these type of medications. That clinic was not put in a medical building. [Jeff George] found a little plaza. You heard about the other businesses that were in the strip shopping center. He brought Theo in and said, 'Theo, my friend, we're going to open up a business. I'm doing another business with my brother, but we're going to open up a business, and we're going to make a lot of money.'

Jeff George also opened up a steroid business. Jeff George is a scoundrel. We asked you during jury selection if you can judge them on what they're saying. He was surrounded by controversy, trouble. He was a smart businessman, and I'll give him that. You saw pictures of the office. Jeff George said, we can open up a pharmacy in the back and make even more money. Ally, a nineteen-year-old girl, ran the pharmacy. They didn't hire a pharmacist.

So now, before they opened, they had to hire a doctor. Jeff George got Dr. Klein's resume. They looked it over and decided to bring him in. They talked to Dr. Klein. They met, and they talked. We know some of the things they talked about were on Dr. Klein's resume. Jeff George's concern was, is the doctor willing to write prescriptions? So that question was asked. Are you willing to write prescriptions that we want you to write?

Yes. No medical background for either Theo Obermeyer or Jeff George. We have an owner telling a doctor what to prescribe.

They were talking about Roxicodone. You see this quantity 240 here and a line to quantity 180. These are the medications that "they" like. Who are they? When you are legitimately seeing patients for pain, you heard all the experts, whether for the State or the defense. They all said the care should be individualized. So when the discussion was quantity 240, [Dr. Klein] didn't put the brakes on. Wait a minute, I'm the doctor. We now know that the line was put there by Gerald Klein, because he said I'm more comfortable prescribing 180. We know that from the first meeting, it wasn't about the well being of the patient. It was about how much to prescribe. When these people came in, they were given packets to fill out. These are the documents that were in the packet, when the patient came in. I'll defer to this as advertising the kinds of drugs they could get and how many.

Initial Packet

OxyContin	80mg	30
Roxicodone	30mg	240
Xanax	2mg	60
Valium	10mg	60
Soma		60

If you recall the questions and arguing between Jeff George and Theo: If someone comes in from the government, and they're suspicious, we'll just blame the doctor. We know in some cases when pharmacy records didn't reconcile, they blamed the doctor. The doctor can point the finger at the patient. Dr. Warfield said drug dealers—those are the people in alleys and streets. Those are the drug dealers. When you open a business and from the first day attract customers. We're not going to take insurance. Cash only. Pharmacy, cash or credit card. When you open up a business like that you are no different than a drug dealer.

We'll make it look legitimate. A facade. Customers would come. Word would get out. And it did. We know that from Alejandro Pino. We heard a lot about the standard of care. Just following the standards, that's not enough. Was [Dr. Klein] conducting a legitimate medical clinic? Was he taking care of the patient? Not if, when a patient wasn't getting the amount they wanted, 240 pills, they would go to the phone and call Jeff George. We know that from Jeff George. Theo and the doctor who left the clinic were both witnesses here. Theo told you when a patient complained, he would talk to Dr. Klein. They would void or tear up the prescription and rewrite it.

Dr. Klein was working part time, three days a week, and making $4,200 a week. That's $218,400 a year. Not bad, for a part time job. And you were told he wanted more money. He wanted $200 an hour. He was told see more patients, write more prescriptions, make the customers happy. He didn't leave. Dr. Klein worked there from the day it opened until the day the DEA closed it down. You heard from Dr. Jones, "I graduated and was looking for a job." He said it didn't take him long to figure it out. "Even I got yelled at if I spent too much time with patients." To the question did you continue to write prescriptions, he answered, "Yes. I was making a lot of money." Dr. Jones left after eight months.

Now, the judge gave you the instructions: Count one felony murder, first degree. Joseph Bartolucci is dead. Trafficking hydromorphone. Gerald Klein caused [that] death, and you know that [Joseph Bartolucci] died from the prescription written by Dr. Klein. The proof is on the bottle that you saw. A picture was taken of it at the residence.

In order to convict, it is not necessary that there was premeditation. I want to explain "deliberate." If the prescription was written, and you find that the doctors who testified are credible, then you can surmise that the prescription was not written in good faith. They told you that there was no medical necessity. This was not a legitimate business.

DEFENSE CLOSING ARGUMENT: SAM RABIN

This is my last opportunity to talk to you. I am not going to summarize the whole trial. There are two tragedies involved: first, death; second, the arrest of Dr. Klein.

Mrs. Bartolucci contacted the prosecutor's office. She was very angry, and I understand that. They can bring charges, and [Dr. Klein] has to sit here. But it has to get through you before you can find that he committed any drug-trafficking offense. As Dr. Warfield pointed out to you, there's high standards and low standards. What I say to you or Ms. Burns says to you is not evidence. I'm going to show you evidence that there was no conspiracy here.

Jeff George taught people what to say. He didn't tell Dr. Klein that he told people what to say. He didn't tell Theo, either. Theo Obermeyer tried to run a legitimate clinic. Do you remember what Theo said? He felt used by Jeff George? They had a sophisticated system at East Coast. Theo stole pills, too. Can't really keep track of the inventory if someone is messing with the numbers. The reason why they had to argue with Dr. Klein is because he was not in on the conspiracy. Dr. Klein said that every patient is different. And that was confirmed by Theo and George.

[Prosecutor Burns] talked about what despicable people they are. But she's letting them testify to reduce their sentence. Do you remember the testimony that when Dr. Klein was told to see patients quicker, he ignored it? He would not bend if the patient was doctor shopping. They were out. He wouldn't see out-of-state patients. They were making Dr. Jones see out-of-state patients. That's why he left. But Dr. Klein refused to see them. What did he tell Mr. Bartolucci? "You shouldn't be taking these oxys"? He told Chris Hutson, "I'm going to wean you."

Let's talk about the rest of the charges. In order for you to find guilty on any of these charges, it has to be an offense. It's not sufficient if it fell out of the standard of care. A lot of witnesses are getting immunity. Come talk to us, and we'll get you out of jail. Come talk to us and we won't report you to the DOH. Ally [Ruiz] came to testify and got nothing in return. She stated: Dr. Klein reviewed the file first. After reviewing the file, he came out and got the patient. Dr. Klein is the only one who would get the file.

Alejandro Pino and Chris Hutson, they couldn't remember anything. You're going to believe someone like that?

They must have remembered enough that the defense attorney doesn't want the jury to believe Pino's and Hutson's testimony. This tactic has worked well for drug companies for years. Accuse the person who became addicted, rather than the one who ensures the pills stay on the market at all costs. It's like blaming a girl for being raped, rather than the aggressor who committed the act.

DEFENSE: There was a discussion with Alejandro Pino about CARP. He told Dr. Klein, "I don't have a drug problem. The only reason I went there was so I could get custody of my kids."

"Custody of my kids"! Alejandro Pino left East Coast Pain on February 26, 2009, with 230 oxycodone 30 mg and 90 Xanax 2 mg. What about the children?

DEFENSE: East Coast is not on trial. Jeff George, Theo, not on trial. They're on their way out the door. Only you can stop that. Chris Hutson, he had an MRI with a very serious problem. He went in and told Dr. Klein, "I'm taking 240 oxycodones. Dr. Klein cut him down to 210. He came in for the second visit, and what does Dr. Klein do? He cuts him down again. Mr. Pino had a terrible accident. He had real pain. Dr. Klein keeps the same 240 oxycodone and takes away OxyContin altogether. And remember, this is a man who had serious pain.

Let me talk about the investigation by Chief Investigator Frazier. First of all, he did not document his work in this case. We also know he tried to get the ME to change her finding from an accidental death to a homicide. He never investigated the numbers on Mr. Bartolucci's phone. Wouldn't that be important? He could have been buying more hydromorphone. They never looked at [Joseph Bartolucci's] girlfriend's phone, either. She said he would borrow her phone and talk secretly. He might have used her phone to make drug deals. But we'll never know. It wasn't investigated.

Dr. Carol Warfield has traveled the world with her work in pain management. The closest the prosecutor's expert witness Dr. Rubenstein would have ever gotten to Harvard would have been to buy a T-shirt.

PROSECUTOR: Objection.

Attorney Rabin may have a future in stand-up comedy if being a trial lawyer doesn't work out.

DEFENSE: Dr. Rubenstein came here with an agenda. Did you see the way he acted on cross exam? He acted pissed. Dr. Carol Warfield, she's written more papers than Dr. Rubenstein has hairs on his head. Dr. Gerber, to me, was the most interesting of all. We didn't find him. He was brought in by the DOH. And the prosecution asks him, on cross exam, if he went to the pain clinic. Her expert witness only reviewed the file, and that's all that was necessary.

I am going to tread lightly. I honestly don't know if Mr. Bartolucci committed suicide, any more than the State can tell you he didn't. He was drug seeking. We know he was thrown out of drug rehab. We know that his best friend gave him a job and then fired him. We know he had a fight with his girlfriend, and she was ending their relationship. He was going home to a mother who loved him very much. We don't have an issue with that. All of these events certainly point to a man who had a lot of problems in his life.

Dr. Warfield, she created the field of pain management. She wrote the book. She said that the medications that Dr. Klein used were appropriate. I have another forty-five minutes, and I'm not using it. I think you get it. I've given you my view.

One thing that I do agree with the defense attorney is that there are two tragedies here. The death of Joseph Bartolucci and the first degree murder trial of this doctor. Although, over the years, I have seen the pain and suffering of parents who will never get over the loss of their child, whatever the outcome here, this is a tragedy for our country. This man on trial for murder has probably never committed another crime in his life.

"Lead us not into temptation and deliver us from evil." The climate was ripe for wrong deeds going unnoticed. A pain clinic could not do business without a doctor's participation. Perhaps, in this case, a good person got caught up in the greed. But I feel a deep compassion in my heart for all of the mothers and fathers who have buried a child. We cannot forget their losses.

The people in attendance at the trial were largely Dr. Klein's family and supporters. While we wait for the jury's decision, I think about Dr. Klein's family. His wife is a lovely woman. The first day I attended the trial, I saw her in the ladies' room. She told me I had gone into her lucky stall, so I always left that one for her on future trips.

THE VERDICT

The jury's verdict on the first-degree murder charge was Not Guilty. The same was found for most of all the other charges. All except one. Doctor Klein was found guilty of selling Xanax to Alejandro Pino. Judge Karen Miller ordered deputies to take Dr. Klein into custody. However, sentencing for Dr. Klein was delayed. The charge could be punishable by up to five years in prison. The defense attorneys requested Judge Karen Miller remove herself from the case due to her prejudicial behavior against Dr. Klein and his attorneys. The decision whether to recuse the judge went as far as the Florida Attorney General's Office. However, Judge Miller was allowed to remain on the case for sentencing.

On March 11, 2016, Dr. Gerald Klein appeared in court to be sentenced for his crime. He first apologized for his mistake. He said he was truly sorry and admitted to making a poor decision in working at the clinic. Rather than prison time, Judge Miller sentenced Dr. Klein to probation and community service.

EPILOGUE

While I end this book before there is any end in sight to the opiate epidemic, in the year since Dr. Klein's trial, there have been some measures put into place that might eventually lead to a better outcome, and I will detail those here.

On Tuesday, March 15, 2016, I checked my emails over morning coffee, as I usually do, and then started my rosary. I often felt like David fighting Goliath, so when I prayed, I asked for help from above. When I finished my morning prayers around 10:30 a.m. and looked at my phone for any new messages before starting my day, I found an email that had not been there an hour before:

> From: Injury Center (CDC)
>
> Date: March 15, 2016 at 9:08 AM
>
> Subject: SAVE THE TIME: NCIPC Partner Call – Update on CDC Guideline for Prescribing Opioids for Chronic Pain
>
> We invite you to join us on Tuesday, March 15, from 1:00-1:45 p.m. on a conference call for an update on CDC's Guideline for Prescribing Opioids for Chronic Pain.

A phone number and code was included. I was so excited that the CDC was instituting guidelines for physicians to follow. Up until then, physicians had been receiving their information regarding oxycodone from the drug companies. Not only did textbooks used in medical schools describe the under-treatment of pain in America, but oxycodone was originally marketed by the drug companies as safe when taken as prescribed. Both of these notions are false, of course. And according to that email, it seemed that the CDC was going to step in and help make a much-needed difference in the way opiates are prescribed in this country.

The phone call was taking place in two-and-a-half hours, which presented a little bit of a challenge. Because, despite my commitment to end the opiate epidemic, I do strive to set time aside for some normalcy in my life, and on that day, I was finally going for a much-needed visit to my hairdresser—but I could not miss that call.

I left early and was able to place myself in my hairdresser, Brian's, chair for the scheduled call at 1:00 p.m. Brian, knew all about the pill mills and my protests. He personally knows people who were affected by the epidemic and had often observed long lines in front of pill mills while driving to his salon. Brian assured me that being on the call would not present a problem for him, and he proceeded to work around my Apple earphones. Thank you, Stencel.

The call started with an introduction to the CDC team, which had diligently researched the need for physician guidelines. As they spoke in turn, each team member presented the facts, explaining how they were striving for the best outcome, while acknowledging that both those suffering from pain and those suffering from the effects of prescription opiates needed to be considered. They discussed the benefits and harm of these drugs.

We all knew, however, the guidelines would not be universally welcomed. Drug companies have a history of responding adversely to any changes that might decrease drug sales. The CDC injury team took great pains (no pun intended) to make sure their research was comprehensive and thorough enough to guard against the blowback that would surely ensue from the chronic pain community.

The rationale and strategies the team employed are quite extensive. You will find the twelve recommended guidelines in Appendix A of this book, along with a link to the forty-one-page document that was presented during the phone call.

That night, still exuberant from the phone call and the events I so hoped could change things, I sent an email to the CDC team regarding the guidelines:

From: Stoppnow@yahoo.com
Sent: Tuesday, March 15, 2016
To: Kinzie (CDC)
Subject: CDC Guidelines

I wanted to thank your team again. Prayers have been answered. I will continue to pray for you as I know you are going to take a lot of heat for this. Know that you did the right thing. Those opposed are being paid for their stance. I also want to thank you for inviting me to hear your announcement.

Sincerely,
Janet Colbert
Founder/President STOPPNow

The next day, I received this reply:

From: Kinzie (CDC)
Subject: RE: CDC Guidelines
Date: March 16, 2016
To: Stoppnow@yahoo.com

Dear Janet:

Thank you so much for your kind note. I can assure you that all of us here at CDC feel the weight of the many lives lost and all potential lives to be saved in embarking on this work. Yesterday was just the beginning, as now the real work begins—ensuring that the Guideline is moved to implementation.

Warm regards,

Kinzie

As the CDC call was taking place, an article was published on MEDPAGE TODAY in which Tom Frieden, Director of the CDC, addressed the media regarding the CDC guidelines.

MEDPAGE TODAY by Kristina Fiore, March 15, 2016

CDC Comes Down Hard on Opioids for Chronic Pain – Urges physicians not to use opioids first-line for chronic pain.

The guidance, although voluntary, is perhaps the strongest federal statement on opioids to date, a step taken to help stop the bleeding from the nation's opioid crises.

"Put simply, the risks of opioids are overdose and death, and the benefits are transient and generally unproven," Tom Frieden, M.D., MPH, director of the CDC, said, during a press briefing. "The epidemic of opioid overdose deaths is doctor-driven, and it can be reversed in part by doctors' actions."

I saw Dr. Frieden speak at the National Drug Summit in Atlanta, Georgia, in 2011. He declared at that time that the incidence of prescription drug overdoses in the United States is epidemic. And in this statement, he once again potentially risked his position to bring this epidemic to the attention of others and to rectify what has resulted from ignoring the problem. To my mind, in taking such a public stance on a controversial topic, Dr. Frieden was acting as a true leader.

Unfortunately, even with these guidelines, doctors are still not required to implement the guidelines. As Dr. Frieden stated, "the guidance [is] voluntary," and the CDC has no power to enact the guidelines as law. While the guidelines do educate physicians in the responsible prescribing of opiates so they no longer need to rely on drug companies as their source of information, we must have legislation to solve the problem. The legislation that would result in fewer pills being prescribed, which would curtail the number of new addictions occurring, requires the support of politicians.

Many addictions start in an acute setting. During Dr. Gerald Klein's trial, witness Alejandro Pino reported that he had been in a bad car accident and did, initially, require relief from his suffering. His treatment, however, should not have resulted, as it did, in an opiate addiction. CDC Guideline #6 addresses this dilemma, and tells physicians that:

> Long-term opioid use often begins with treatment of acute pain. When opioids are used for acute pain, clinicians should prescribe the lowest effective dose of immediate-release opioids and should prescribe no greater quantity than needed for the expected duration of pain severe enough to require opioids. Three days or less will often be sufficient; more than seven days will rarely be needed.

Many people have told me that even a trip to the dentist has resulted in an inordinate number of pills being prescribed, rather than what would be sufficient for one or two days, at which point, the patient could switch to an anti-inflammatory medication. However, you can refuse oxycodone, when it is offered. Remember, it is not just kids who have made a bad decision and are dying. So keep yourself and family members safe: Tell your doctor or dentist that you do not need an opiate for treatment, unless it is absolutely necessary.

The number of opioid-related deaths for those aged forty-five to fifty-four years continues to increase. The CDC reported, in the **Morbidity and Mortality Weekly Report** (MMWR) on January 1, 2016:

> Opioid pain reliever prescribing has quadrupled since 1999 and has increased in parallel with overdoses involving the most commonly used opioid pain relievers.

Now, in 2016, we face a resurgence of heroin deaths throughout the country that starts with the prescription pain pill (heroin and oxycodone are both opiates). Eight out of ten heroin addicts start with oxycodone. The subsequent heroin epidemic has caused an escalation of new HIV cases. It's a pebble thrown into a stream that continues to ripple.

The drug companies got us into this mess; they employed the doctors to do their dirty work. I have spoken to many legislators, both at the state and national level, who are content to maintain the status quo. There is no urgency for our elected officials to do anything to stop the deaths. In fact, the drug lobbyists are the biggest lobbyists.

Perhaps, then, the answer lies in the increasing roar from our local communities. The United Way of Broward County organized an Advocacy Action Team, as well as a Community Response Team in an effort to address the over prescribing of oxycodone. I am a part of both teams. We are very blessed to have Jim Hall, an epidemiologist at Nova Southeastern University, as an active participant in these meetings. Jim has a wealth of knowledge and has spoken to congressional committees on a state and national level, yet he is the humblest man I know. He shares the most current statistics of the opiate epidemic with our groups and is passionate about finding solutions.

Local law enforcement is actively involved in the meetings, as well. Law enforcement representatives have discussed the balance between the financial cost to the community if first responders carry Narcan (an antagonist for the opiate administered to an overdose victim) and the human cost if they do not carry it. For instance, the young man who died in Joy's home while she administered CPR could have been saved with Narcan. Instead, another mother grieves.

The medical examiner is often present at the meetings. Some of those who attend come from centers that are actively involved with the suffering of those trying to become clean. Bobbie Linkhorn, from South Florida Wellness Network, reported that there were three deaths in Broward County Rehab Centers just a week before I wrote this, including a mother found dead on a bathroom floor, by her children, a needle still in her arm.

We would like to see needle exchange programs, Narcan carried by first responders, and more rehab beds. But my top priority is to have fewer pills prescribed. Whether we are mothers or law enforcement officers, each one of us brings our piece of the puzzle, in hopes that together we can stop the escalation of opioid-related deaths.

More than fifty years ago, the then U.S. Surgeon General sought to reveal the role of "Big Tobacco" in tobacco-related illnesses and death. Like the opioid-producing drug companies today, the tobacco companies hid the addictive nature of tobacco. But as a result of the Surgeon General's campaign, eventually, public service announcements warning of the dangers of tobacco use were broadcast, warning labels were placed on cigarette packages, and advertisements to promote cigarettes were stopped. The result was that nearly half of adult smokers quit.

I have often wondered where our current U.S. Surgeon General is regarding the opiate epidemic. I attended the Fed-Up Rally in Washington, D.C., in October 2015. The next day, on the National Mall, the group Unite to Face Addiction held a large rally. I've heard reports that 10,000 people attended. I was there, and I just know it was a lot. A woman who came to the rally from Alaska told me she liked my STOPPNow shirt. She also shared that her daughter had become addicted and was now serving time in prison for her role in the prescription drug epidemic. That mother embodies the issue of love for one's child, whose life is forever ruined by opiate use.

I got to hear the U.S. Surgeon General, Vivek Murthy, speak. His speech was so uplifting. He announced that he would be releasing the first-ever Surgeon General's Report on substance use, addiction, and health in the early months of 2016. It seemed that help was on the way.

My husband and I made our way through the crowds on the mall, toward the metro station. I saw the Surgeon General on the sidewalk waiting for his car. I introduced myself and told him about STOPPNow, the drug addicted babies I was caring for, and all the parents I have met along the way who have buried their children. When I told him I was from Broward County, Florida, he said that he went to high school in Miami and thanked me for what I am doing. Some of the people with him seemed to be his family members, and one of them asked if I would like him to take my picture with the Surgeon General. Of course, I was delighted. He was such a down-to-earth, sincere man.

Almost one year after our meeting on the sidewalk on the National Mall, the U.S. Surgeon General has acted. In an unprecedented move, on August 27, 2016, he sent a letter to every physician in the United States. The title reads, *U.S. Surgeon General's Call to End the Opioid Crisis*, and in it he states opioids were strongly marketed to doctors, many of whom were taught incorrectly

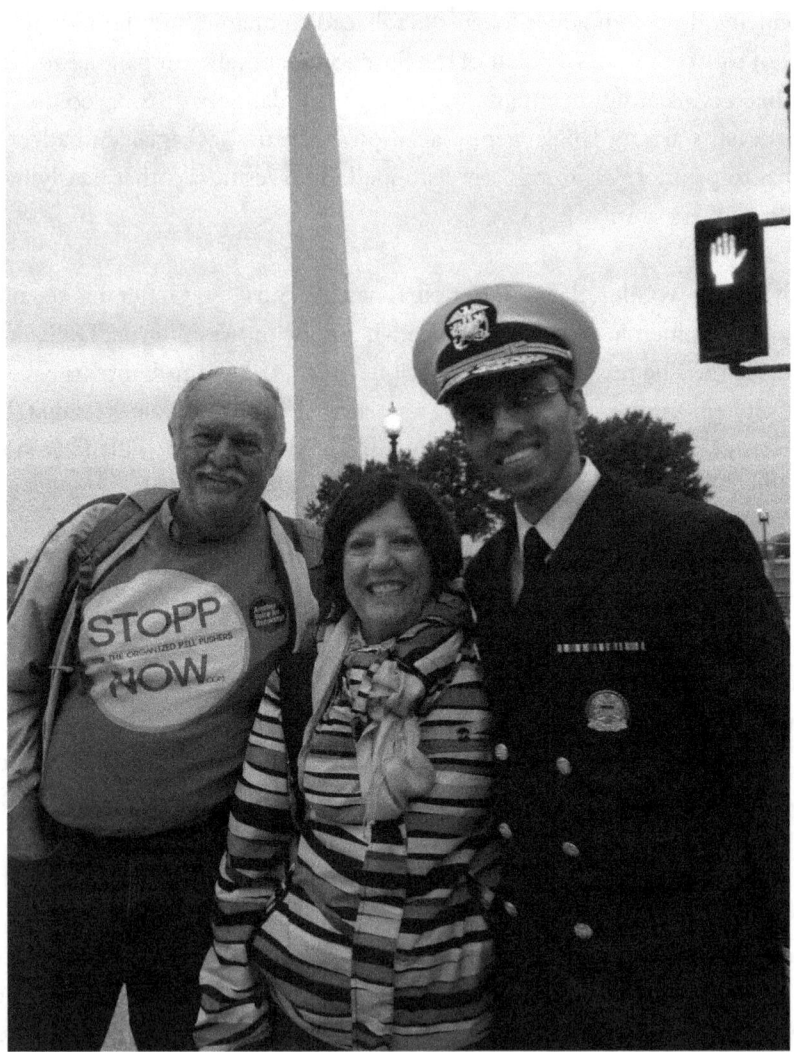

Robert and Janet Colbert of STOPPNow with U.S. Surgeon General Vivek Murthey. Washington Monument in the background.

that opioids are not addictive when prescribed for legitimate pain. Embedded in the letter is a pocket guide for physicians to follow. In the guideline, in all capital letters, it states: IN GENERAL, DO NOT PRESCRIBE OPIOIDS AS THE FIRST LINE TREATMENT FOR CHRONIC PAIN. The Surgeon General does exclude active cancer care and palliative or end of life care from this guideline. He also says, *For acute pain, prescribe less than a three-day supply.* (You can find the complete letter at http://turnthetiderx.org and in Appendix B of this book.)

During my years of fighting to alleviate the opiate epidemic my hopes have often been raised, only to be extinguished. This was the case with both the International Drug Caucus and the so-called Senate Investigation. No arrests have been made and there have been no effective changes as a result of either. After the Surgeon General's letter was disseminated, I decided to follow up with Senator Feinstein's office, and wrote an email to Kelly Lieupo, who is associated with Senator Feinstein's office, in regards to Drug Caucus matters.

> From: Janet Colbert stoppnow@yahoo.com
> Subject: Opiate Deaths
> Date: September 2, 2016 10:51 AM
> To: Lieupo, Kelly (Feinstein)
>
> Kelly:
>
> I have not heard back from you. I'm sure you and Senator Feinstein are aware of the U.S. Surgeon General's letter to all physicians in the United States. I am still interested to know if Senator Feinstein is investigating the corruption involved and if she has received an answer to the letters sent by her and Senator Grassley? If you are not familiar with the letter sent by the Surgeon General or the referral card, they can be found on stoppnow.com website.
>
> Sincerely,
> Janet Colbert
> Founder/President STOPPNow

I received a response the same day:

> From: Kelly Lieupo
> To: STOPPNow
> Re: Opiate Deaths
>
> Janet:
>
> Thanks for your email, and I apologize for the delay in my response.

Yes, we are aware of the Surgeon General's recent actions related to the opioid epidemic and the letter he sent to all physicians, which was a positive step. You may also be interested to know that HHS announced $53 million in grants this week to help combat this epidemic.

As far as the issue with Purdue is concerned, as you pointed out in 2014, my boss, along with other members of the Drug Caucus, sent letters to Purdue and others regarding the "region zero" database allegedly maintained by the company, which, according to the *LA Times*, contained information about doctors overprescribing OxyContin. Following this, it was revealed that in many cases, neither the Drug Enforcement Administration, state medical boards, or the Centers for Medicare and Medicaid Services were aware of this database. Senators Feinstein and Grassley encouraged these organizations to contact Purdue about the database, which they did, and they gained access to the pertinent information.

Should you have any additional questions, please let me know.

Thanks,
Kelly

I replied.

To: Kelly Lieupo
Re: Opiate Deaths

Kelly:

Yes, the *LA Times* has been able to uncover a lot. I wish they had arrest power. We need legislation that would result in fewer pills. We can't just keep throwing money at it. Let's end it.

Janet

The chairman of the International Drug Caucus, Senator Feinstein, seems content with forwarding the *L.A. Times* report over to the DEA, state medical boards, and Centers for Medicare and Medicaid Services. And their job is done. The rate of opioid overdoses has tripled since 2000, and this is their answer?

Watergate started with an investigative report by Bob Woodward and Carl Bernstein of the *Washington Post*. The difference is that the Senate in the 1970s saw the need to investigate Watergate further. They were not content to let it end with the *Washington Post* exposing a story. I hope we never lose the free press in our country. It is also up to us, the people, to make sure our legislators do not become apathetic. Or have they already?

On September 22, 2016, I attended a Heroin and Opioid Awareness Town Hall meeting in Boca Raton, Florida. The town hall meeting was presented by the United States Attorney's Office. The problem is, of course, getting worse. I was interested in attending because there was hope that we would be seeing "the big guns" become involved in combating the opiate epidemic. About two weeks prior to the Town Hall meeting, a controversial picture was released by the East Liverpool Police Department in Ohio. The picture was of a man and a woman passed out in a car with a baby strapped into a car seat in the back of the vehicle. The police department was criticized for releasing the picture. But this is what is happening in our streets. We can't blame the messenger for pointing out the truth. Blame our legislators, instead, for the prescription drug situation being allowed to spiral out of control due to their inaction.

A similar incident was reported in Miami. And Emily, the mother in Louisville, Kentucky, that I spoke of earlier, noticed a girl slumped over the driver's seat in a car next to her at a traffic light. Emily got out of her car, opened the door, and found the girl unconscious with drug paraphernalia beside her on the front seat. Emily called 911, and they were able to revive the girl with Narcan. Emily saved someone else's child that day, yet, she still suffers every day from the loss of her own. Emily now carries Narcan in the glove compartment of her car.

In addition to this unsafe maelstrom taking place on our streets, I have read reports of librarians who carry Narcan in their pockets who have revived overdose victims in the library, also not an isolated incident.

With all of this information occupying my thoughts, I trudged up to Boca Raton for the Town Hall Meeting on Heroin and Opioid Awareness. I never give up. Something might change. While I am aware that the Caucus on International Narcotics Control, featuring Chairman Senator Feinstein and Senator Chuck Grassley (coming to a theatre near you) expressing their true concern and commitment, has not resulted in one less pill being produced, still, I was hopeful.

Unfortunately, there were not any legislators present at the town hall meeting.

Disturbing facts were presented at the meeting, however. Medical examiners reported the increase in drug-related deaths they are seeing. Jim Hall informed those in attendance of the latest available data. He stated that due to there not being a system in place for real-time reporting, this is a "barefoot epidemiology" from the medical examiners' offices (confirmed in this meeting as well) by medical examiners from numerous counties, health care administration, and hospitals.

2015

Southern Region of Florida Opiate deaths (oxycodone, heroin, fentanyl)

Miami Dade County: 478 opiate overdose deaths.

972 non-fatal (reversed with Narcan)

Broward County: 367 opiate overdose deaths.

732 non-fatal (reversed with Narcan)

Palm Beach County: 412 deaths

818 non-fatal (reversed with Narcan)

Monroe County: 74 overdoses

Five counties to the north: 527 overdoses

In the Southern Region of Florida, a conservative number of overdoses is reported as 4,380 (non-fatal), with 1,460 deaths in 2015. That is an opiate death every six hours (four per day), as well as an overdose every two hours – or twelve overdoses per day in the Southern Region of Florida alone.

As horrible as these statistics are, the medical examiners reported that, so far in 2016, they are seeing double that amount. Jim Hall reported the finding as a "ninety-one percent increase in deaths for the year 2016." We won't know the total insult until late 2017, when the numbers have been conclusively calculated.

There are twenty-four medical examiner districts in the state of Florida, covering sixty-seven counties. The data collection for 2015 was released in September, 2016. Below, are highlights from the Medical Examiner (ME) Report for 2015 for the State of Florida.

> Total drug-related deaths increased by 13.9 percent (1,197) when compared with 2014.

> 5,364 (an increase of 12.4 percent compared with 2014) individuals died with one or more prescription drugs in their system. The drugs were identified as either the cause of death or merely present in the decedent. These drugs may have also been mixed with illicit drugs and/or alcohol.

> 2,530 (an increase of 22.7 percent compared with 2014) individuals died with at least one prescription drug in their system that was identified as the cause of death. These drugs may have been mixed with other prescription drugs, illicit drugs, and/or alcohol.

> Prescription drugs (benzodiazepines, carisoprodol/meprobamate, zolpidem, and all opioids excluding heroin) continued to be found more often than illicit drugs, both as the cause of death and present at death. **Prescription drugs account for 67.7 percent of all drug occurrences in this report when ethyl alcohol is excluded.**

> Occurrences of heroin increased by 74.3 percent and deaths caused by heroin increased by 79.7 percent when compared with 2014.

> **Occurrences of oxycodone increased by 10.5 percent and deaths caused by oxycodone increased by 20.2 percent when compared with 2014.**

The entire fifty-nine-page report can be viewed on this link: http://www.fdle.state.fl.us/cms/MEC/Publications-and-Forms/Documents/Drugs-in-Deceased-Persons/2015-Annual-Drug-Report.aspx

The U. S. Surgeon General's Report promised for release by the beginning of 2016, which can be found at https://addiction.surgeongeneral.gov, was released November 17, 2016. The report states that the number of drug-related deaths in 2014 was higher than in any previous year on record: *In 2014, there were 47,055 drug overdose deaths including 28,647 people who died from a drug overdose involving some type of opioid, including prescription pain relievers and heroin.*

The monetary cost is noted as well: *Substance misuse and substance use disorders also have serious economic consequences costing more than $400 billion annually in crime, health, and lost productivity.* The need for more and better treatment is also examined: *Only about one in ten people with a substance use disorder receive any type of specialty treatment.* And, in Chapter 2 of the report, mention is made of studies regarding the path opiates travel through the brain, changing the brain chemistry of the user along the way.

Finally, I'd like to note this from the report: *Well-supported scientific evidence shows that medications can be effective in treating serious substance use disorders, but they are under-used. The U.S. Food and Drug Administration (FDA) has approved three medications to treat alcohol use disorders and three others to treat opioid use disorders.*

So, the FDA, which is well aware of the problems caused by the opiate, continues to approve more opiates and then the Medically Assisted Treatment (MAT) necessary to treat the addiction caused by the opiate. And the drug companies make money on both ends: First, by causing the addiction, and then by treating it.

Therefore, while I am disappointed that the report does not demand the production of the opiate be either halted altogether or markedly reduced, I am not surprised. Nor am I surprised that there is no mention in the report of the role drug companies' marketing of this extremely dangerous drug to the public and the way they incentivize doctors to prescribe it.

Overall, I find the U.S. Surgeon's Report to be too broad. The inclusion of alcohol and other addictive chemicals dissipates the focus on the opiate epidemic and impedes a direct route to the solution to end that epidemic. In the chapter relating to prevention the Surgeon General notes, *In the early 1980s, President Ronald Reagan established a bipartisan presidential commission to reduce drunk driving. The commission's first recommended action was to raise the Minimum Legal Drinking Age to twenty-one.* The report also refers to Mothers Against Drunk Driving (MADD) getting legislation to support this measure. MADD was started by a mother after the death of her child due to drunk driving.

There is no mention in the report, however, of the fact that in 1984 President Reagan signed into law legislation banning domestic production and sales of the prescription drug Quaalude. To enforce this law, the DEA first shut down manufacturers of methaqualone powder (needed to produce Quaaludes) in foreign countries. This is an example of what can happen when the DEA is allowed to do its job. Quaaludes were also legal prescription drugs, in this case prescribed by doctors for insomnia. The production of Quaaludes was banned because of the number of deaths the drug caused—which is small, compared to the deaths caused by prescription opiates.

While Broward County, Florida, is considered the epicenter of the opiate epidemic, its effects are felt in every state in our country. The CDC posts statistics that confirm that the deaths and devastation continue to rise each year. And yet no state has instituted the CDC's guidelines into law—and the FDA continues to approve new opiates. Other drugs that cause more harm than good have been removed from the market. Why not oxycodone?

Each one of us has a different gift to bring to the table and help fight this fight. Get mad. Get active. Get on the phone. Write a letter. This freight train must be stopped. Now.

Janet Colbert
Founder STOPPNow
and Michael

Unless someone like you cares a whole awful lot, nothing is going to get better. It's not.
– Dr. Seuss, *The Lorax*

APPENDIX A

CDC Guideline for Prescribing Opioids for Chronic Pain, 2016

For complete forty-one-page report, see
http://dx.doi.org/10.15585/mmwr.rr6501e1er

1. Nonpharmacological therapy and nonopioid pharmacologic therapy are preferred for chronic pain. Clinicians should consider opioid therapy only if expected benefits for both pain and function are anticipated to outweigh risks to the patient. If opioids are used, they should be combined with nonpharmacologic therapy and nonopioid pharmacologic therapy, as appropriate

2. Before starting opioid therapy for chronic pain, clinicians should establish treatment goals with all patients, including realistic goals for pain and function, and should consider how opioid therapy will be discontinued if benefits do not outweigh risks. Clinicians should continue opioid therapy only if there is clinically meaningful improvement in pain and function that outweighs risks to patient safety

3. Before starting and periodically during opioid therapy, clinicians should discuss with patients known risks and realistic benefits of opioid therapy and patient and clinician responsibilities for managing therapy

4. When starting opioid therapy for chronic pain, clinicians should prescribe immediate-release opioids instead of extended-release/long-acting (ER/LA) opioids

5. When opioids are started, clinicians should prescribe the lowest effective dosage. Clinicians should use caution when prescribing opioids at any dosage, should carefully reassess evidence of individual benefits and risks when considering increasing dosage to ≥50 morphine milligram equivalents (MME)/day, and should avoid increasing dosage to ≥90 MME/day or carefully justify a decision to titrate dosage to ≥90 MME/day

6. Long-term opioid use often begins with treatment of acute pain. When opioids are used for acute pain, clinicians should prescribe the lowest effective dose of immediate-release opioids and should prescribe no greater quantity than needed for the expected duration of pain severe enough to require opioids. Three days or less will often be sufficient; more than seven days will rarely be needed

7. Clinicians should evaluate benefits and harms with patients within one to four weeks of starting opioid therapy for chronic pain or of dose escalation. Clinicians should evaluate benefits and harms of continued therapy with patients every three months or more frequently. If benefits do not outweigh harms of continued opioid therapy, clinicians should optimize other therapies and work with patients to taper opioids to lower dosages or to taper and discontinue opioids

8. Before starting and periodically during continuation of opioid therapy, clinicians should evaluate risk factors for opioid-related harms. Clinicians should incorporate into the management plan strategies to mitigate risk, including considering offering naloxone when factors that increase risk for opioid overdose, such as history of overdose, history of substance use disorder, higher opioid dosages (≥50 MME/day), or concurrent benzodiazepine use, are present

9. Clinicians should review the patient's history of controlled substance prescriptions using state prescription drug monitoring program (PDMP) data to determine whether the patient is receiving opioid dosages or dangerous combinations that put him or her at high risk for overdose. Clinicians should review PDMP data when starting opioid therapy for chronic pain and periodically during opioid therapy for chronic pain, ranging from every prescription to every three months

10. When prescribing opioids for chronic pain, clinicians should use urine drug testing before starting opioid therapy and consider urine drug testing at least annually to assess for prescribed medications as well as other controlled prescription drugs and illicit drugs

11. Clinicians should avoid prescribing opioid pain medication and benzodiazepines concurrently whenever possible

12. Clinicians should offer or arrange evidence-based treatment (usually medication-assisted treatment with buprenorphine or methadone in combination with behavioral therapies) for patients with opioid use disorder.

APPENDIX B

Letter from The U.S. Surgeon General

Dear Colleague:

I am asking for your help to solve an urgent health crisis facing America: the opioid epidemic. Everywhere I travel, I see communities devastated by opioid overdoses. I meet families too ashamed to seek treatment for addiction. And I will never forget my own patient whose opioid use disorder began with a course of morphine after a routine procedure.

It is important to recognize that we arrived at this place on a path paved with good intentions. Nearly two decades ago, we were encouraged to be more aggressive about treating pain, often without enough training and support to do so safely. This coincided with heavy marketing of opioids to doctors. Many of us were even taught – incorrectly – that opioids are not addictive when prescribed for legitimate pain.

The results have been devastating. Since 1999, opioid overdose deaths have quadrupled and opioid prescriptions have increased markedly – almost enough for every adult in America to have a bottle of pills. Yet the amount of pain reported by Americans has not changed. Now, nearly two million people in America have a prescription opioid use disorder, contributing to increased heroin use and the spread of HIV and hepatitis C.

I know solving this problem will not be easy. We often struggle to balance reducing our patients' pain with increasing their risk of opioid addiction. But, as clinicians, we have the unique power to help end this epidemic. As cynical as times may seem, the public still looks to our profession for hope during difficult moments. This is one of those times.

That is why I am asking you to pledge your commitment to turn the tide on the opioid crisis. Please take the pledge. Together, we will build a national movement of clinicians to do three things: First, we will educate ourselves to treat pain safely and effectively. A good place to start is the TurnTheTideRx pocket guide with the CDC Opioid Prescribing Guideline. Second, we will screen our patients for opioid use disorder and provide or connect them with evidence-based treatment. Third, we can shape how the rest of the country sees addiction by talking about and treating it as a chronic illness, not a moral failing.

Years from now, I want us to look back and know that, in the face of a crisis that threatened our nation, it was our profession that stepped up and led the way. I know we can succeed because health care is more than an occupation to us. It is a calling rooted in empathy, science, and service to humanity. These values unite us. They remain our greatest strength.

Thank you for your leadership.

Vivek H. Murthy, M.D., M.B.A.

19th U.S. Surgeon General

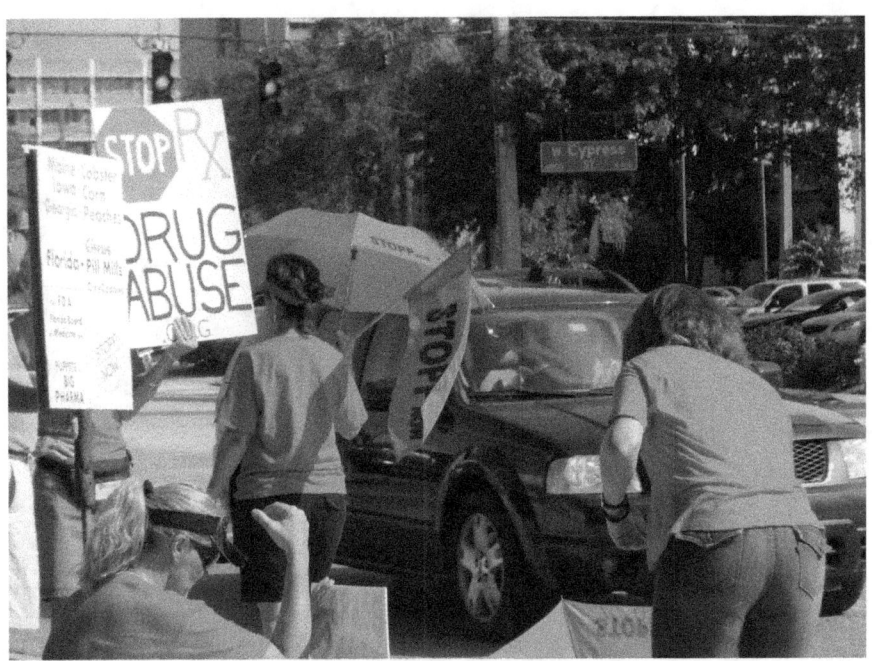
Tampa BOM protest.

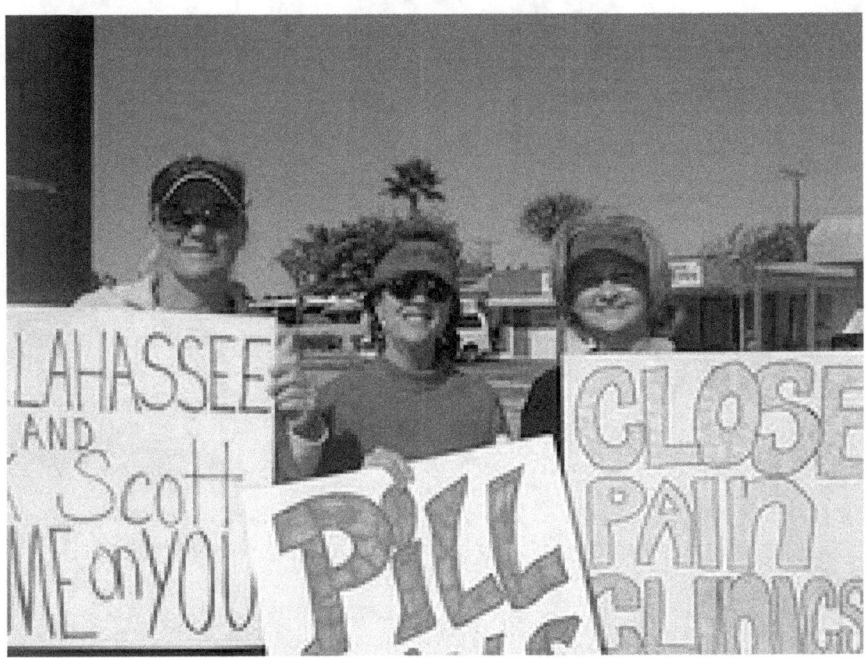
Joy, Janet, Renee. Vincent Colangelo's "PILL MILL"

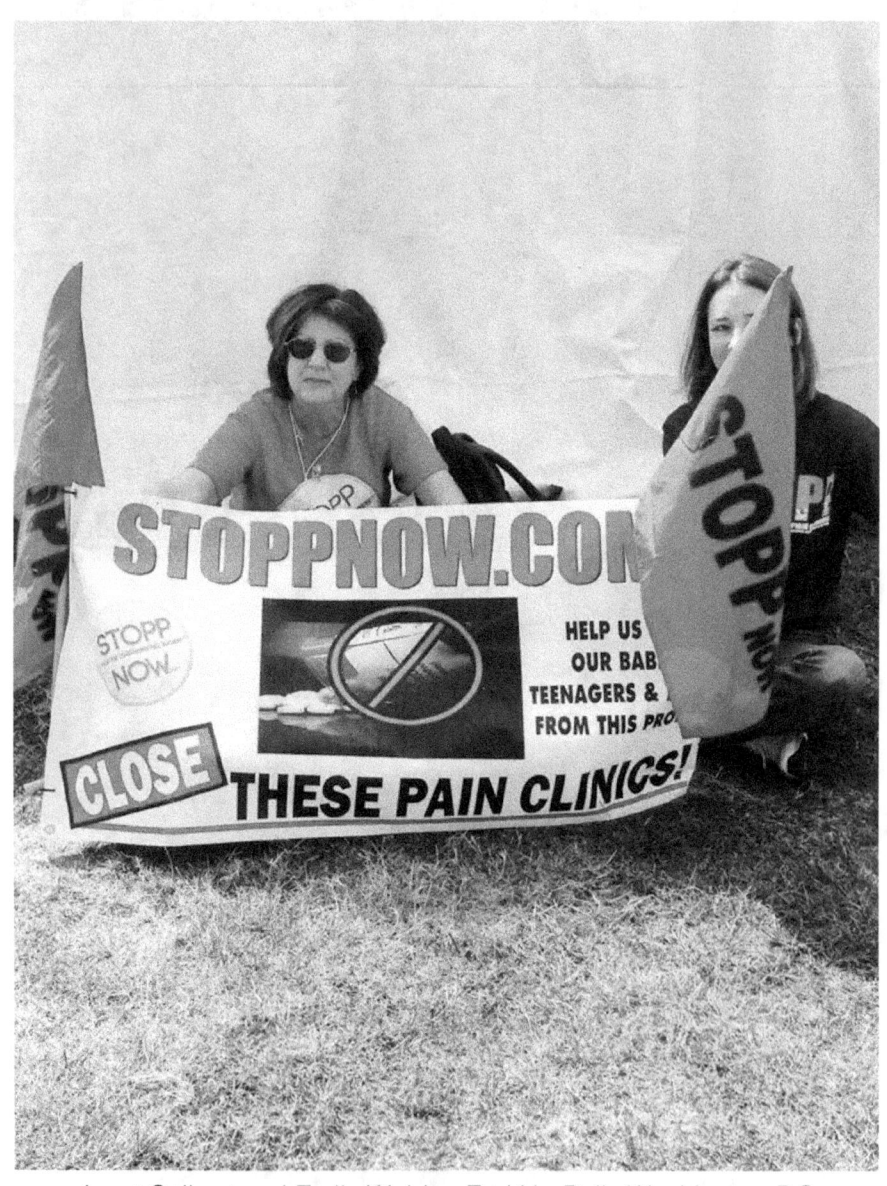

Janet Colbert and Emily Walden Fed Up Rally Washington DC

www.ingramcontent.com/pod-product-compliance
Lightning Source LLC
Chambersburg PA
CBHW071012200526
45171CB00007B/13